FREE Test Taking Tips DVD Offer

To help us better serve you, we have developed a Test Taking Tips DVD that we would like to give you for FREE. **This DVD covers world-class test taking tips that you can use to be even more successful when you are taking your test.**

All that we ask is that you email us your feedback about your study guide. Please let us know what you thought about it – whether that is good, bad or indifferent.

To get your **FREE Test Taking Tips DVD**, email freedvd@studyguideteam.com with "FREE DVD" in the subject line and the following information in the body of the email:

   a. The title of your study guide.

   b. Your product rating on a scale of 1-5, with 5 being the highest rating.

   c. Your feedback about the study guide. What did you think of it?

   d. Your full name and shipping address to send your free DVD.

If you have any questions or concerns, please don't hesitate to contact us at freedvd@studyguideteam.com.

Thanks again!

Adult CCRN Study Guide 2020 & 2021

Adult CCRN Review Book & Practice Exam Questions [3rd Edition Prep]

Test Prep Books

Interested in buying more than 10 copies of our product? Contact us about bulk discounts:
bulkorders@studyguideteam.com

ISBN 13: 9781628457674
ISBN 10: 1628457678

Table of Contents

Quick Overview

As you draw closer to taking your exam, effective preparation becomes more and more important. Thankfully, you have this study guide to help you get ready. Use this guide to help keep your studying on track and refer to it often.

This study guide contains several key sections that will help you be successful on your exam. The guide contains tips for what you should do the night before and the day of the test. Also included are test-taking tips. Knowing the right information is not always enough. Many well-prepared test takers struggle with exams. These tips will help equip you to accurately read, assess, and answer test questions.

A large part of the guide is devoted to showing you what content to expect on the exam and to helping you better understand that content. In this guide are practice test questions so that you can see how well you have grasped the content. Then, answer explanations are provided so that you can understand why you missed certain questions.

Don't try to cram the night before you take your exam. This is not a wise strategy for a few reasons. First, your retention of the information will be low. Your time would be better used by reviewing information you already know rather than trying to learn a lot of new information. Second, you will likely become stressed as you try to gain a large amount of knowledge in a short amount of time. Third, you will be depriving yourself of sleep. So be sure to go to bed at a reasonable time the night before. Being well-rested helps you focus and remain calm.

Be sure to eat a substantial breakfast the morning of the exam. If you are taking the exam in the afternoon, be sure to have a good lunch as well. Being hungry is distracting and can make it difficult to focus. You have hopefully spent lots of time preparing for the exam. Don't let an empty stomach get in the way of success!

When travelling to the testing center, leave earlier than needed. That way, you have a buffer in case you experience any delays. This will help you remain calm and will keep you from missing your appointment time at the testing center.

Be sure to pace yourself during the exam. Don't try to rush through the exam. There is no need to risk performing poorly on the exam just so you can leave the testing center early. Allow yourself to use all of the allotted time if needed.

Remain positive while taking the exam even if you feel like you are performing poorly. Thinking about the content you should have mastered will not help you perform better on the exam.

Once the exam is complete, take some time to relax. Even if you feel that you need to take the exam again, you will be well served by some down time before you begin studying again. It's often easier to convince yourself to study if you know that it will come with a reward!

Test-Taking Strategies

1. Predicting the Answer

When you feel confident in your preparation for a multiple-choice test, try predicting the answer before reading the answer choices. This is especially useful on questions that test objective factual knowledge. By predicting the answer before reading the available choices, you eliminate the possibility that you will be distracted or led astray by an incorrect answer choice. You will feel more confident in your selection if you read the question, predict the answer, and then find your prediction among the answer choices. After using this strategy, be sure to still read all of the answer choices carefully and completely. If you feel unprepared, you should not attempt to predict the answers. This would be a waste of time and an opportunity for your mind to wander in the wrong direction.

2. Reading the Whole Question

Too often, test takers scan a multiple-choice question, recognize a few familiar words, and immediately jump to the answer choices. Test authors are aware of this common impatience, and they will sometimes prey upon it. For instance, a test author might subtly turn the question into a negative, or he or she might redirect the focus of the question right at the end. The only way to avoid falling into these traps is to read the entirety of the question carefully before reading the answer choices.

3. Looking for Wrong Answers

Long and complicated multiple-choice questions can be intimidating. One way to simplify a difficult multiple-choice question is to eliminate all of the answer choices that are clearly wrong. In most sets of answers, there will be at least one selection that can be dismissed right away. If the test is administered on paper, the test taker could draw a line through it to indicate that it may be ignored; otherwise, the test taker will have to perform this operation mentally or on scratch paper. In either case, once the obviously incorrect answers have been eliminated, the remaining choices may be considered. Sometimes identifying the clearly wrong answers will give the test taker some information about the correct answer. For instance, if one of the remaining answer choices is a direct opposite of one of the eliminated answer choices, it may well be the correct answer. The opposite of obviously wrong is obviously right! Of course, this is not always the case. Some answers are obviously incorrect simply because they are irrelevant to the question being asked. Still, identifying and eliminating some incorrect answer choices is a good way to simplify a multiple-choice question.

4. Don't Overanalyze

Anxious test takers often overanalyze questions. When you are nervous, your brain will often run wild, causing you to make associations and discover clues that don't actually exist. If you feel that this may be a problem for you, do whatever you can to slow down during the test. Try taking a deep breath or counting to ten. As you read and consider the question, restrict yourself to the particular words used by the author. Avoid thought tangents about what the author *really* meant, or what he or she was *trying* to say. The only things that matter on a multiple-choice test are the words that are actually in the question. You must avoid reading too much into a multiple-choice question, or supposing that the writer meant something other than what he or she wrote.

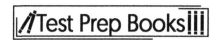

5. No Need for Panic

It is wise to learn as many strategies as possible before taking a multiple-choice test, but it is likely that you will come across a few questions for which you simply don't know the answer. In this situation, avoid panicking. Because most multiple-choice tests include dozens of questions, the relative value of a single wrong answer is small. As much as possible, you should compartmentalize each question on a multiple-choice test. In other words, you should not allow your feelings about one question to affect your success on the others. When you find a question that you either don't understand or don't know how to answer, just take a deep breath and do your best. Read the entire question slowly and carefully. Try rephrasing the question a couple of different ways. Then, read all of the answer choices carefully. After eliminating obviously wrong answers, make a selection and move on to the next question.

6. Confusing Answer Choices

When working on a difficult multiple-choice question, there may be a tendency to focus on the answer choices that are the easiest to understand. Many people, whether consciously or not, gravitate to the answer choices that require the least concentration, knowledge, and memory. This is a mistake. When you come across an answer choice that is confusing, you should give it extra attention. A question might be confusing because you do not know the subject matter to which it refers. If this is the case, don't eliminate the answer before you have affirmatively settled on another. When you come across an answer choice of this type, set it aside as you look at the remaining choices. If you can confidently assert that one of the other choices is correct, you can leave the confusing answer aside. Otherwise, you will need to take a moment to try to better understand the confusing answer choice. Rephrasing is one way to tease out the sense of a confusing answer choice.

7. Your First Instinct

Many people struggle with multiple-choice tests because they overthink the questions. If you have studied sufficiently for the test, you should be prepared to trust your first instinct once you have carefully and completely read the question and all of the answer choices. There is a great deal of research suggesting that the mind can come to the correct conclusion very quickly once it has obtained all of the relevant information. At times, it may seem to you as if your intuition is working faster even than your reasoning mind. This may in fact be true. The knowledge you obtain while studying may be retrieved from your subconscious before you have a chance to work out the associations that support it. Verify your instinct by working out the reasons that it should be trusted.

8. Key Words

Many test takers struggle with multiple-choice questions because they have poor reading comprehension skills. Quickly reading and understanding a multiple-choice question requires a mixture of skill and experience. To help with this, try jotting down a few key words and phrases on a piece of scrap paper. Doing this concentrates the process of reading and forces the mind to weigh the relative importance of the question's parts. In selecting words and phrases to write down, the test taker thinks about the question more deeply and carefully. This is especially true for multiple-choice questions that are preceded by a long prompt.

9. Subtle Negatives

One of the oldest tricks in the multiple-choice test writer's book is to subtly reverse the meaning of a question with a word like *not* or *except*. If you are not paying attention to each word in the question, you can easily be led astray by this trick. For instance, a common question format is, "Which of the following is…?" Obviously, if the question instead is, "Which of the following is not…?," then the answer will be quite different. Even worse, the test makers are aware of the potential for this mistake and will include one answer choice that would be correct if the question were not negated or reversed. A test taker who misses the reversal will find what he or she believes to be a correct answer and will be so confident that he or she will fail to reread the question and discover the original error. The only way to avoid this is to practice a wide variety of multiple-choice questions and to pay close attention to each and every word.

10. Reading Every Answer Choice

It may seem obvious, but you should always read every one of the answer choices! Too many test takers fall into the habit of scanning the question and assuming that they understand the question because they recognize a few key words. From there, they pick the first answer choice that answers the question they believe they have read. Test takers who read all of the answer choices might discover that one of the latter answer choices is actually *more* correct. Moreover, reading all of the answer choices can remind you of facts related to the question that can help you arrive at the correct answer. Sometimes, a misstatement or incorrect detail in one of the latter answer choices will trigger your memory of the subject and will enable you to find the right answer. Failing to read all of the answer choices is like not reading all of the items on a restaurant menu: you might miss out on the perfect choice.

11. Spot the Hedges

One of the keys to success on multiple-choice tests is paying close attention to every word. This is never truer than with words like almost, most, some, and sometimes. These words are called "hedges" because they indicate that a statement is not totally true or not true in every place and time. An absolute statement will contain no hedges, but in many subjects, the answers are not always straightforward or absolute. There are always exceptions to the rules in these subjects. For this reason, you should favor those multiple-choice questions that contain hedging language. The presence of qualifying words indicates that the author is taking special care with his or her words, which is certainly important when composing the right answer. After all, there are many ways to be wrong, but there is only one way to be right! For this reason, it is wise to avoid answers that are absolute when taking a multiple-choice test. An absolute answer is one that says things are either all one way or all another. They often include words like *every*, *always*, *best*, and *never*. If you are taking a multiple-choice test in a subject that doesn't lend itself to absolute answers, be on your guard if you see any of these words.

12. Long Answers

In many subject areas, the answers are not simple. As already mentioned, the right answer often requires hedges. Another common feature of the answers to a complex or subjective question are qualifying clauses, which are groups of words that subtly modify the meaning of the sentence. If the question or answer choice describes a rule to which there are exceptions or the subject matter is complicated, ambiguous, or confusing, the correct answer will require many words in order to be expressed clearly and accurately. In essence, you should not be deterred by answer choices that seem excessively long. Oftentimes, the author of the text will not be able to write the correct answer without offering some qualifications and modifications. Your job is to read the answer choices thoroughly and completely and to select the one that most accurately and precisely answers the question.

13. Restating to Understand

Sometimes, a question on a multiple-choice test is difficult not because of what it asks but because of how it is written. If this is the case, restate the question or answer choice in different words. This process serves a couple of important purposes. First, it forces you to concentrate on the core of the question. In order to rephrase the question accurately, you have to understand it well. Rephrasing the question will concentrate your mind on the key words and ideas. Second, it will present the information to your mind in a fresh way. This process may trigger your memory and render some useful scrap of information picked up while studying.

14. True Statements

Sometimes an answer choice will be true in itself, but it does not answer the question. This is one of the main reasons why it is essential to read the question carefully and completely before proceeding to the answer choices. Too often, test takers skip ahead to the answer choices and look for true statements. Having found one of these, they are content to select it without reference to the question above. Obviously, this provides an easy way for test makers to play tricks. The savvy test taker will always read the entire question before turning to the answer choices. Then, having settled on a correct answer choice, he or she will refer to the original question and ensure that the selected answer is relevant. The mistake of choosing a correct-but-irrelevant answer choice is especially common on questions related to specific pieces of objective knowledge. A prepared test taker will have a wealth of factual knowledge at his or her disposal, and should not be careless in its application.

15. No Patterns

One of the more dangerous ideas that circulates about multiple-choice tests is that the correct answers tend to fall into patterns. These erroneous ideas range from a belief that B and C are the most common right answers, to the idea that an unprepared test-taker should answer "A-B-A-C-A-D-A-B-A." It cannot be emphasized enough that pattern-seeking of this type is exactly the WRONG way to approach a multiple-choice test. To begin with, it is highly unlikely that the test maker will plot the correct answers according to some predetermined pattern. The questions are scrambled and delivered in a random order. Furthermore, even if the test maker was following a pattern in the assignation of correct answers, there is no reason why the test taker would know which pattern he or she was using. Any attempt to discern a pattern in the answer choices is a waste of time and a distraction from the real work of taking the test. A test taker would be much better served by extra preparation before the test than by reliance on a pattern in the answers.

FREE DVD OFFER

Don't forget that doing well on your exam includes both understanding the test content and understanding how to use what you know to do well on the test. We offer a completely FREE Test Taking Tips DVD that covers world class test taking tips that you can use to be even more successful when you are taking your test.

All that we ask is that you email us your feedback about your study guide. To get your **FREE Test Taking Tips DVD**, email freedvd@studyguideteam.com with "FREE DVD" in the subject line and the following information in the body of the email:

- The title of your study guide.
- Your product rating on a scale of 1-5, with 5 being the highest rating.
- Your feedback about the study guide. What did you think of it?
- Your full name and shipping address to send your free DVD.

Introduction to the Adult CCRN Exam

Function of the Exam

The Adult Acute/Critical Care Nursing Certification (CCRN®) exam is required to obtain the CCRN specialty certification, which is one of several specialty certifications offered to nurses by the AACN Certification Corporation. Nurses who work in settings where they provide direct care to adult, pediatric, or neonatal patients needing acute or critical care can seek CCRN® certification, which demonstrates competency in the knowledge and skills needed for their job, as well as professional recognition of their commitment to the field, their careers, and the care of acutely/critically ill patients. Accordingly, CCRN® test takers are nurses who typically work in intensive care units, combined ICU/CCUs, trauma units, cardiac care units, medical/surgical ICUs, or in critical care transport. CCRN® nurses need to deliver high-intensity, specialized care to their patients with a high degree of vigilance. Care may be focused on a specific system, such as renal, cardiac, or pulmonary, or it may be more generalized, geared toward multisystem, systemic issues.

The CCRN® exams are designed based on a job analysis, which examines the practice and skills of registered nurses (RNs) or advanced practice registered nurses (APRNs) who provide direct care to adult, pediatric, or neonatal patients who are acutely/critically ill. This process occurs at least every five years and helps determine and validate the abilities, skills, and knowledge needed to work with one of these patient populations in situations where the patients are acutely/critically ill. An expert CCRN® panel then works to ensure the exams are designed to reflect the findings of the job analysis and clinical practice. There is a separate exam for each patient population—adult, pediatric, and neonatal—and candidates should select the exam that best reflects the primary patient population for whom they provide direct care.

Exam candidates must have a current, unencumbered RN or APRN license from the United States. Additionally, one of the following two clinical practice requirements must be met prior to sitting for the exam:

- At least 1,750 hours providing direct care to acutely ill adult patients over the previous two years as an RN or APRN, with at least 875 of those hours obtained in the most recent year

- At least 2,000 hours providing direct care to acutely ill adult patients over the previous five years as an RN or APRN, with at least 144 of those hours obtained in the most recent year

It should be noted that orientation hours do not count towards minimum hour requirements unless the candidate was the assigned nurse who was providing direct care to patients with acute/critical illnesses during those hours.

Test Administration

Candidates can register online or via a paper application for the exam. After receiving an approval-to-test email, they can schedule their exam administration. The email will include a specific 90-day period during which the candidate must schedule and take the exam. The exam is offered twice daily, Monday through Friday, and some Saturdays, at more than 300 PSI/AMP testing locations around the United States. The exam is offered in a computer and paper-and-pencil format. Scores are provided immediately after submitting the computer-based version, and are received three to four weeks after sitting for the paper version. The exam may be retaken for an additional fee.

Test Format

The Adult CCRN® exam, like the pediatric and neonatal versions, contains 150 multiple-choice questions, of which, 125 are scored. The remaining 25, which are randomly scattered throughout the exam, are used to gauge their worth for inclusion in future versions. Test takers are given three hours to complete the exam. Clinical Judgment comprises 80% of the questions while Professional Caring and Ethical Practice topics contribute 20% of the questions. It should be noted that the Clinical Judgment questions pertain only to adult patients, while the Professional Caring and Ethical Practice questions will address patients across the lifespan. The following table provides the domains of the adult version of the exam and the breakdown of their approximate percentage contributions to the total:

Domain	Percentage of Exam*
Clinical Judgment	80%
Cardiovascular	18%
Pulmonary	17%
Endocrine/Hematology/Gastrointestinal/Renal/Integumentary	20%
Musculoskeletal/Neurology/Behavioral	13%
Multisystem	14%
Professional Caring and Ethical Practice	20%

*Note that the percentage of questions from the Clinical Judgement and Professional Caring and Ethical Practice domains are fairly firm at 80% and 20%, respectively. However, the percent contribution of questions pertaining to the specific body systems are approximated and therefore, do not necessarily sum to exactly 80%.

Scoring

A panel of subject matter and exam experts establish the passing score of the Adult CCRN® exam. The passing score is established via the modified Angoff, a criterion-referenced process for setting standards. Each test taker's CCRN® exam performance is compared to the predetermined standard to determine his or her passing status. The difficulty rating of each question also impacts the value of answering a question correctly. The passing score is said to be established to identify those candidates who possess an acceptable level of knowledge and skill in providing care to acutely ill adult patients. Candidates who successfully pass the exam receive a certificate denoting their specialty certification within three to four weeks after passing the test.

Study Prep Plan for the Adult CCRN Exam

1   **Schedule -** Use one of our study schedules below or come up with one of your own.

2   **Relax -** Test anxiety can hurt even the best students. There are many ways to reduce stress. Find the one that works best for you.

3   **Execute -** Once you have a good plan in place, be sure to stick to it.

Sample Study Plans

One Week Study Schedule

Day 1	Clinical Judgment
Day 2	Pulmonary
Day 3	Endocrine/Hemotology/Gastrointestinal/Renal/Integumentary
Day 4	Musculoskeletal/Neurology/Psychosocial
Day 5	Professional Caring & Ethical Practice
Day 6	Practice Questions
Day 7	Take Your Exam!

Two Week Study Schedule

Day 1	Cardiovascular	Day 8	Practice Questions
Day 2	Practice Questions	Day 9	Advocacy/Moral Agency
Day 3	Pulmonary	Day 10	Caring Practices
Day 4	Practice Questions	Day 11	Response to Diversity
Day 5	Endocrine/Hematology/Gastrointestinal/Renal/Integumentary	Day 12	Clinical Inquiry
Day 6	Practice Questions	Day 13	Practice Questions
Day 7	Musculoskeletal/Neurology/Psychosocial	Day 14	Take Your Exam!

One Month Study Schedule							
Day 1	Acute Coronary Syndromes	Day 11	Acute Respiratory Failure	Day 21	Renal/Genitourinary
Day 2	Acute Peripheral Vascular Insufficiency	Day 12	Air-Leak Sydromes	Day 22	Practice Questions
Day 3	Acute Pulmonary Edema	Day 13	Aspiration	Day 23	Musculoskeletal
Day 4	Arterial Venous Occlusion	Day 14	Status Asthmaticus	Day 24	Neurological
Day 5	Cardiac/Vascular Catheterization	Day 15	Thoracic Surgery	Day 25	Practice Questions
Day 6	Cardiomyopathies	Day 16	Thoracic Trauma	Day 26	Advocacy/Moral Agency
Day 7	Dysrythmias	Day 17	Practice Questions	Day 27	Caring Practices
Day 8	Practice Questions	Day 18	Endocrine	Day 28	Response to Diversity
Day 9	Acute Pulmonary Embolus	Day 19	Hematology/ Immunology	Day 29	Practice Questions
Day 10	Acute Respiratory Distress Syndrome (ARDS)	Day 20	Gastrointestinal	Day 30	Take Your Exam!

Clinical Judgment

In the world of patient care, the nurse is the vigilante, always watching and guarding the patient. A continuous series of clinical judgments are made based upon patient assessment, tests, lab work, procedure results, data analysis, and team collaboration. The critical care registered nurse (CCRN) is highly adept at putting together all these pieces of the patient puzzle, making informed clinical judgments that will greatly benefit the patient's care. The following is a review of cardiovascular and pulmonary maladies. The nurse pursuing CCRN certification must be familiar with these conditions, causes, signs and symptoms, and course of treatment to make appropriate clinical judgments regarding the patient's care.

Cardiovascular

The critical care nurse is an expert at recognizing a cardiovascular illness, from the crushing weight felt by a patient with angina, to the classic shooting pain up and down the left arm of a patient experiencing a heart attack, to the pooling of blood in the legs when one's circulatory system has weakened. Savvy knowledge of the cardiovascular system and the different ways it can malfunction is a key factor in a critical care nurse's ability to make sound clinical judgments. The following is a review of acute cardiovascular diseases in critical care settings.

Acute Coronary Syndromes

An acute coronary syndrome is any instance in which the coronary arteries of the heart are blocked, causing an interrupted flow in crucial oxygen delivery to the heart muscle. This causes immediate damage to the areas affected, and if left untreated, tissue death. A more common term for the syndrome, though less precise, is a **heart attack**.

There are three distinct types of acute coronary syndromes: unstable angina, non–ST-segment elevation myocardial infarction (NSTEMI), and STEMI. The latter two refer to what most people know as "heart attacks," differing only by the amount of the heart wall that is damaged. **Angina**, a term for chest pain, can occur without heart tissue damage. All three categories can occur because of increased oxygen demand in the heart tissue or the body at large, such as during exercise and emotional distress.

In any of the three cases, major determining factors for tissue damage include the severity of the arterial blockage, the length of time the arteries are blocked, the percentage of the heart that is affected, the magnitude of the demand for oxygen in the heart, and the extent to which the heart can compensate for the oxygen loss.

A patient may be experiencing a different condition than acute coronary syndrome, such as an anxiety attack or acid reflux, that may mimic the same signs and symptoms. The clinician must be aware of this possibility when making a clinical judgment. An accurate assessment will be made based on patient history, clinical presentation, and events leading up to the current symptoms.

The most common symptom that signals acute coronary syndrome is chest pain. The chest pain of a heart attack has been described as "crushing pressure," "heavy weight," "tightness," and/or "fullness" in the chest area above the heart. Other accompanying symptoms include a shooting pain up and down one or either arm, along the jawline, or even in the back or abdomen. The patient may complain of "not being able to catch their breath," breathing rapidly, with shallow depth of breath. Dizziness, lightheadedness, nausea, and profuse drops of sweat may be part of the patient's presentation.

It is important to note that gender plays a role in how patients may present with a heart attack. Considering that heart disease is the leading cause of death for women in the United States, the critical care nurse should be aware that women may not exhibit the classic signs of a heart attack. A woman is more likely to have non-chest-related symptoms, such as nausea, anxiety, and radiating pain in the upper or lower back and jaw region. These symptoms may occur weeks before the actual attack, making correct diagnosis even more difficult to pinpoint. That being said, knowing that there may be a different presentation will help the critical care nurse make the correct clinical judgment regarding the situation, considering all involved factors.

Acute MI and Myocardial Ischemia

The previous section discussed acute coronary syndromes, STEMIs, and NSTEMIs. This section will expound on the two distinct forms of MI. Diagnosis of MI is made by electrocardiogram (ECG) reading as well as serological markers such as elevated troponin.

Diagram illustrating normal ECG, ST elevation, ST depression, and T inversion

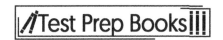

An **NSTEMI** is an MI in which the ST segment of the ECG is not elevated. This important distinction arises from the amount of heart muscle damaged. In an NSTEMI, not enough heart tissue is damaged to make the ST segment rise on the ECG, whereas a STEMI does just that.

Serological markers such as an elevated troponin level indicate cardiac muscle damage. When the muscle is injured, it releases muscle cell contents into the bloodstream; the greater the damage, the higher the muscle cell contents, such as troponin, in the bloodstream. Other serological markers indicating heart muscle damage include the cardiac enzymes CK-MB and muscle cell component myoglobin.

After the ECG has been checked and the blood has been sent to the lab to evaluate for elevated serological markers of a heart attack, the patient will likely be whisked away for a cardiac catheterization. This standard procedure includes accessing the patient's femoral artery, threading a thin tube, or catheter, up through the abdominothoracic blood vessels directly into the heart to assess for blockages and damage. During the test, dye is released into the heart, and x-ray images are obtained for better visualization. The patient will often be given medication to relax, but they will still be awake for the procedure. This procedure can allow the cardiologist to open up coronary vessels that have been occluded with atherosclerotic plaques using a tiny balloon and place tiny metal scaffolds called **stents**, if necessary, and determine if further interventions such as cardiac surgery are needed to repair valves or bypass severely blocked arteries.

Illustration of the thickness of heart muscle affected in the heart wall in NSTEMI vs. STEMI

Transverse section of the heart

Partial thickness damage

Full thickness damage

Illustration of the papillary muscles in the heart

One particularly disastrous complication of an MI is when the **papillary muscles**—five total within the heart—rupture following an attack. These five muscles—three in the right ventricle and two in the left—are attached to the mitral and tricuspid valves, which also known as the **atrioventricular valves** due to their position between the atria and ventricles. Essentially, the infarcted tissue begins to break down, leading to the papillary muscles to fall apart if left untreated for long enough. When they break loose, the atrioventricular valves become dysfunctional, causing an acute valve regurgitation; then fluid collects in the lungs, which causes pulmonary edema, followed promptly by cardiogenic shock and death. Rupture of the papillary muscles is a medical emergency and requires swift treatment to prevent mortality.

Signs that a patient having an MI may be developing papillary muscle rupture include auscultating a loud, apical, holosystolic murmur accompanied by a thrill. The regurgitation may be silent. An

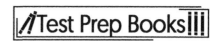

echocardiography test should be run to confirm diagnosis. The patient will likely display dramatic hemodynamic decline such as falling blood pressure (BP), racing heart rate, decreased level of consciousness, difficulty breathing, and poor oxygenation. The patient will need emergency surgery to repair or replace the regurgitating mitral valve.

Acute Peripheral Vascular Insufficiency

There are two types of peripheral vascular insufficiency: venous and arterial. In either case, insufficiency predominantly occurs in the legs rather than the arms because of gravity on the lower portion of the body. This is not to say that arms cannot be affected by vascular insufficiency, but it occurs there more rarely.

Arterial insufficiency can be acute or chronic, and it varies in severity. The more severe the narrowing of the arteries in the extremity, the more profound the symptoms will be. Caused by sclerosis in the arteries of the lower extremities, arterial insufficiency causes pain in the legs, due to a decreased blood flow and thus a decreased delivery of oxygen to the muscle tissue. Other manifestations of an atherosclerotic arterial system are loss of hair; bluish tint, or cyanosis, of the skin; gangrene; and ischemic ulcers.

Treatment for arterial insufficiency includes diet modification, risk factor reduction, exercise, and medications targeted at preventing clots and treating symptoms such as pain. Arterial insufficiency can occur acutely because of a clot.

Diagnosis for peripheral arterial insufficiency is obtained through a comparison of the ankle BP and the brachial BP, called the **ankle-brachial BP index**. Blood vessels will be visualized using ultrasonography as well as angiography if the patient will be going for surgery to correct the issue.

Venous insufficiency occurs when the valves and walls of the venous system weaken and malfunction. The result is pooling of blood in the extremities that would have normally returned to the heart for recirculation. This can be an acute occurrence in the case of volume overload, such as in pregnancy.

Edema caused by venous insufficiency may be accompanied by throbbing, cramping pain along with aches, heaviness, and fatigue of the legs. Risk factors include having a clot in the leg called a **deep vein thrombosis (DVT),** which is the most common cause, as well as obesity, older age, and a direct trauma to the venous vasculature.

Carotid Artery Stenosis

Carotid artery stenosis is a subcategory of peripheral vascular insufficiency involving the arteries of the neck that supply the brain with nutrient-filled blood. This condition may exist long before symptoms occur, as the narrowing may not be severe enough to significantly reduce blood flow to the brain. Stenosis, the narrowing of a blood vessel, in this case is most often caused by **atherosclerosis**. This entails a building up of a fatty substance called **plaque** inside the artery walls, which leads to reduced blood flow.

An acute condition involving carotid artery stenosis is when a clot occurs at the site of the stenosis, interrupting blood flow completely. This leads to a transient ischemic attack (TIA), or worse, a cerebrovascular accident (CVA), commonly referred to as a **stroke**. A TIA is an episode that mimics stroke symptoms, such as slurring of speech, drooping of face, and other neurologic deficits, and lasts for less than an hour but longer than five minutes. There is no long-term damage, as the episode is transient enough that no brain tissue is injured. A TIA may be the first clue the patient has that they have carotid artery stenosis, as there are few to no symptoms beforehand.

Risk factors for developing carotid artery stenosis include alcohol abuse, hypertension, smoking, high cholesterol, diabetes, obesity, stress, heart disease, drug abuse (especially cocaine and amphetamines), vascular inflammation, history of stroke, and old age. Smoking cessation information should be given to the patient to encourage them to quit.

Carotid artery stenosis is diagnosed most commonly with carotid ultrasound, using sonography to visualize the arterial structures in the neck. Other tests that may be ordered include carotid angiography, magnetic resonance angiography, and computerized tomography angiography (CAT).

The arteries may be stented or partially removed to correct the stenosis. Antiplatelet therapy will ensue as well as anticoagulants to prevent future blood clots.

Endarterectomy
The patient with atherosclerosis of the carotid artery may be a candidate for a surgical procedure called an **endarterectomy**. In this surgery, the carotid artery is accessed by a surgeon, incised, and the problematic plaque carefully removed. The artery is then sutured closed, and the patient will likely be sent to an intensive care unit (ICU) to recover.

Endarterectomy

Carotid arteries
Located in the neck

A
Internal carotid artery

Plaque

Common carotid artery

B
Incision (cut) in artery wall

Plaque removed by surgeon

C
Normal blood flow restored

Incision stitched to repair the artery

Narrow artery cross-section

Palque

Reduce blood flow

Narrow artery cross-section

Normal blood flow restored

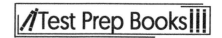

The critical care nurse will be carefully monitoring the patient in the hours and days following the surgery. Since a major artery was accessed, bleeding is the first and most obvious complication to be monitored for. The incision site will be monitored not only for signs of becoming infected, but for hematoma or signs of bleeding. There may be wound drains for which patency needs to be maintained. The patient must be taught to support their head with their hands when moving to minimize strain of the neck muscles. Clots are still a threat to this patient's well-being, so the nurse will monitor for any signs that the carotid artery has become occluded again or that the patient is experiencing a CVA. Signs of a CVA include sudden onset of neurologic deficits such as confusion, dizziness, slurred speech, or paralysis of the arms and/or legs.

Hemodynamic monitoring, already a standard practice in the ICU, will be critical to determine if the patient is developing complications. Hypotension could indicate volume loss or possibly lead to myocardial ischemia. Hypertension puts the patient at risk of developing a CVA, as well as putting added pressure on the recently incised and healing artery.

The critical care nurse will monitor for signs of respiratory distress, such as a change in rate, rhythm, depth, and effort of breath. The nurse will also be mindful of tracheal deviation from the midline and patient restlessness, as well as difficulty swallowing. These could be signs of excessive swelling and could lead to further respiratory distress. It is recommended that a patient who has had an endarterectomy have a tracheostomy kit at their bedside, in case of an emergency.

The patient will likely be put on antiplatelet therapy in the post-op period, including aspirin at 100 mg daily and clopidogrel at 75 mg daily for at least the first thirty days, starting day one post-op. A major complication in the post-operative period is clotting and/or restenosis of the artery, and this therapy aims to prevent that.

Femoropopliteal Bypass

A femoropopliteal (fem-pop) bypass graft is a surgical procedure that reroutes blood in the leg past an occluded section of artery, caused by atherosclerosis. The patient's own vein may be used, or an artificial vein will be used, though this presents a risk for narrowing over time. The vein bypasses the occlusion starting at the femoral artery and ending at the popliteal artery in the knee.

Femoropopliteal Bypass

This procedure is used for patients with severe claudication. ***Claudication*** is a word of Latin origin, originally meaning "limp," but in this case, it means severe pain in the legs caused by restricted blood supply. Claudication may occur in the feet or, most commonly, in the calves. The patient may also be experiencing sores that will not heal or gangrene due to restricted blood flow. The bypass will reinstate healthy blood flow to previously ischemic areas, hopefully alleviating symptoms.

Patients should be encouraged to quit smoking before the procedure to prevent complications and promote overall health. Smoking cessation information and resources should be shared early and often.

Patients will be anesthetized for the procedure. Blood transfusion is a distinct possibility to maintain volume and replace blood loss. The incision made by the surgeon is generally 4 to 8 inches in length, in the groin area where the femoral artery is located. Internal stitches will be made to secure the graft in place. The patient may be in surgery anywhere from 1 to 6 hours depending on the complexity of the surgery.

The nurse in the critical care unit receiving the patient postop will want to monitor the incision site for infection, bleeding, and/or hematoma. Hemodynamic monitoring will be in place to watch for hypotension, which could indicate bleeding, or hypertension, which could put added pressure on the

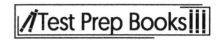

healing graft. Like postoperative therapy for a carotid endarterectomy, the patient will be put on antiplatelet and antithrombotic therapy to prevent clotting and restenosis of the vessels.

Peripheral Stents

Peripheral stents are another option to attempt to open occluded arteries in a patient with peripheral arterial disease (PAD). Stent placement occurs at the same time as angioplasty, in which a small thin catheter is threaded into the affected blood vessel, and a tiny balloon is inflated to "pop" open the lumen of the blood vessel. Then, stent placement can occur.

The stent is usually a tiny metal, mesh-like tube that provides a scaffolding or support structure to keep a blood vessel open. The stent remains in the patient's blood vessel permanently, although it is possible to remove a stent if absolutely necessary.

Antiplatelet and antithrombotic therapies will be used in the post-operative period.

Acute Pulmonary Edema

When there is disease and dysfunction in the heart and circulatory system, one of the first systems of the body to be affected is the pulmonary system. The lungs have an intimate relationship with the function of the heart, and when the heart is no longer pumping effectively or the blood vessels are no longer circulating the blood efficiently throughout the body, the lungs bear the brunt of it. **Cardiogenic** is a term that refers to a condition originating in or caused by the heart.

One condition caused by the heart that affects the lungs is cardiogenic pulmonary edema. When the heart fails to pump effectively, the pulmonary venous pressure rises. Remember that the pulmonary vein is the vein of the heart that carries oxygenated blood from the lungs back to the left atrium of the heart after gas exchange in the pulmonary capillaries. When this pressure rises, fluid begins to build up in the lungs.

There are many different reasons fluid can build up in the lungs in addition to this example, such as an imbalance of Starling forces, alveolar–capillary barrier damage, an obstruction of lymphatic circulation, or even of an idiopathic nature. The critical care nurse will recall that the Starling forces entail the Starling equation, in which hydrostatic and oncotic forces work together to move fluid across a capillary membrane, as in the case of oxygen exchange in the alveolar beds of the lungs.

The patient with pulmonary edema will be given supplemental oxygen therapy, diuretics to decrease volume load, and heart medication, depending on their condition. Preload in the heart will be targeted, using diuretics such as furosemide (Lasix®) or nifedipine (Procardia®). If shortness of breath and anxiety are severe, as is the case sometimes, morphine may be prescribed to lessen oxygen demand. The patient may be prescribed agents to reduce afterload, such as nitroprusside, which will cause dilation of the coronary arteries, relieving pressure in the hardworking left ventricle. Blood pressure will be used according to the patient's history and clinical presentation, maintaining a normal pressure for optimal blood flow.

The patient experiencing pulmonary edema may have changes in respiratory patterns and decreased oxygenation. The labor of breathing may worsen, increasing fatigue. The patient may require assisted or mechanical ventilation if the condition deteriorates into respiratory distress and failure, until the pulmonary edema has resolved, per the attending physician's discretion.

Arterial Venous Occlusion

When an artery or vein is blocked by a clot, this occlusion is termed a **thrombosis**. Clot formation is a normal hemostatic adjustment that occurs in a healthy individual to prevent excessive bleeding and promote wound healing. Inappropriate clotting, however, can interrupt critical blood flow, and thus oxygen delivery to the tissues of the body. Interruption in oxygen delivery, if not corrected, will lead to tissue damage and death.

Occlusion of an artery may sometimes occur because of atherosclerosis, in which fatty deposits called **plaques** build up over time, sticking to the walls of the vessels. These fatty deposits are composed of lipids, inflamed smooth muscle cells, and a connective tissue matrix composed of thrombi in various stages, as well as calcium deposits.

A person may not know that they have atherosclerosis until a plaque bursts or occludes blood flow, causing ischemic conditions such as stroke or heart attack.

Persons who smoke should be encouraged to cease, as smoking is one of the greatest risk factors for developing atherosclerosis. Nicotine and other chemicals found in cigarette or cigar smoke are toxic to the inner lining of blood vessels. These toxins inflame and scar the vascular endothelium, not only increasing the risk of plaque accumulation, but also causing vasoconstriction. Vasoconstriction in already narrowed blood vessels increases BP and puts the smoker in danger of other life-threatening events such as clots and IAs.

Other risk factors for atherosclerosis include high cholesterol, diabetes, family history, sedentary lifestyle, obesity, and high BP.

To confirm a diagnosis of atherosclerosis, the affected blood vessels need to be visualized by imaging techniques such as angiography or ultrasonography.

Modifications in lifestyle such as diet, exercise, and smoking cessation will be encouraged for the patient with atherosclerosis. Drug therapy will include antiplatelets such as aspirin at 100 mg daily and statins for targeting lipids such as atorvastatin at 40–80 mg per day.

A common venous occlusion is a DVT. Though DVTs may be asymptomatic, the common presentation is redness, pain, and swelling over the site of the clot. Common sites for DVT are the lower extremities, specifically the superficial femoral, popliteal, posterior tibial, or peroneal veins in the calves. DVTs come about because of impaired venous return, an injury to the endothelium such as leg fractures, or in states of hypercoagulability in which the body is more apt to make clots. Impaired venous return is common in immobile patients. Therefore, early ambulation is encouraged as well as mobility exercises while the patient is still in bed, to prevent clots.

DVTs in the lower extremities have a high correlation with patients also developing pulmonary embolisms (PEs), or blood clots that travel to the lungs. This is a life-threatening situation and will be discussed in detail in a subsequent section. Other complications of DVTs include a chronic insufficiency of the veins and post-phlebitic syndrome, in which a patient feels aching, cramping, pain, and other symptoms in the legs that worsen with walking or standing and are relieved by resting.

A D-dimer is the test used to help diagnose a DVT. A negative result rules out a DVT, while a positive is not 100 percent conclusive. A positive d-dimer necessitates further testing—usually ultrasonography—

to confirm the diagnosis. History and physical examination are also helpful in determining the probability of a DVT.

If left untreated, there is a high likelihood that the patient with a DVT will develop a PE and die; therefore, detection and treatment are vital. Treatment is usually with anticoagulants such as subcutaneous heparin for a short period followed by a longer period of oral warfarin. Pain control with nonsteroidal anti-inflammatory drugs (NSAIDs) may be included in the treatment plan, along with leg elevation with pillows while the patient is at rest, being careful to avoid venous compression, which could lead to clot dislodgement.

Peripheral Vascular Insufficiency

Some patients may suffer with chronic insufficiencies of the peripheral vascular system, both arterial and venous.

PAD is a chronic condition in which the arteries of the extremities—almost always lower extremities—are narrowed and sometimes blocked by atherosclerotic plaques. This causes ischemia, in which vital oxygen delivery is interrupted and tissue damage and death occurs. Symptoms of PAD include claudication, wounds or ulcers that will not heal, cyanosis of the extremity, loss of hair in the extremity, and atrophy of the skin. Treatment is usually with lifestyle modifications including smoking cessation, and drug therapy including antiplatelets such as aspirin or cilostazol.

Chronic venous insufficiencies occur when the veins' ability to return blood to the heart is impaired. This disease also occurs more frequently in the lower extremities because of gravity. The cause of this insufficiency usually arises from immobility, in which lack of muscle contraction surrounding the veins leads to vein weakness and dysfunction. Another cause is venous hypertension, which usually occurs after a DVT. Symptoms of chronic venous insufficiencies include a feeling of fullness or heaviness in the legs, aching, cramping, and fluid accumulation, or edema. Treatment includes elevation of the affected limb(s), compression to encourage flow, and treatment of a secondary infection, if present.

Patients with chronic venous insufficiency are at high risk for developing venous stasis ulcers. Areas where blood has pooled are vulnerable to injury, followed by wounds that will not heal due to poor circulation.

Both patients with venous and arterial insufficiencies are prone to these types of nonhealing ulcers. A differentiating factor between venous and arterial ulcers is that venous are usually superficial and arterial are deeper, eventually exposing deep fascia such as tendons and bones. Adequate care of lower extremities in both cases of venous and arterial insufficiencies is vital to prevent secondary infections.

Cardiac/Vascular Catheterization

A critical care nurse is well-acquainted with the cardiac catheterization procedure, as it is such a powerful and common tool to determine if a patient has cardiac disease. As discussed earlier, the test involves the threading of a small, thin catheter through peripheral arteries or veins up to the heart, obtaining information about the chambers, valves, and structures therein, the pulmonary artery, the coronary arteries, and the veins.

There are two different approaches to cardiac catheterization: left heart and right heart. If the cardiologist wishes to access the left heart, commonly to determine anatomy of the heart, BP in the aorta, or to assess aortic or mitral valve function, they will access the femoral artery and enter the heart through the aorta on the left side. For left heart catheterization, the subclavian, radial, or brachial arteries may also be accessed, but less commonly.

For right heart catheterization, the venous system is accessed. The heart is approached from the right side, entering through the right atrium where venous blood is returning. Right heart cardiac catheterization is used to determine the pressures in the right atria, right ventricle, and pulmonary arteries, as well as the pulmonary artery occlusion pressure (PAOP). Common venous access sites used for right heart catheterization are the femoral, subclavian, internal jugular, or antecubital veins.

The method of visualization used in cardiac catheterization is through the injection of radiopaque contrast into the heart chambers and surrounding structures while x-ray images are taken to produce images. This is called **angiography**. Another visualization technique uses tiny ultrasound transducers placed at the end of the catheter to produce images. Angiography and ultrasonography can be used at the same time.

Patients with kidney disease may not be good candidates for undergoing a cardiac catheterization due to the contrast that is used. When this dye is shot into the heart, it must be metabolized by the kidneys, which in a damaged kidney, could lead to further damage. Patients with active infections, fever, heart failure, heart arrhythmias, and coagulopathies may also be poor candidates for cardiac catheterizations, at the discretion of the physician.

To prepare for a cardiac catheterization, the patient will be kept nil per os (NPO) for 4 to 6 hours pre-catheterization. During the procedure, the patient will be given medication to help them relax, but will not be put under general anesthesia.

Diagnostic

There are two uses for cardiac catheterization: diagnostic and interventional. The diagnostic approach means the cardiologist is looking to assess the anatomy of the heart and determine its functioning ability. Disease states will be evaluated. Common diagnostic uses of cardiac catheterization include angiography, intravascular ultrasonography, measuring of cardiac output, biopsy of tissues within the heart, shunt detection, and measurement of the heart's metabolic function.

Interventional

The second approach to cardiac catheterization is interventional, often occurring during a diagnostic procedure. A problem is seen, and action is taken to correct it. Common interventions during cardiac catheterization are percutaneous transluminal coronary angioplasty and stent insertion.

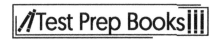

The tip of the cardiac catheter is a tiny balloon that can be inflated to open occluded arteries, a procedure termed **angioplasty.** After balloon inflation, the cardiologist may choose to insert a stent into the reopened artery to maintain patency of the vessel. Stent placement is used often in the case of acute MI. This intervention helps restore blood flow to areas of ischemia in the heart following a coronary artery occlusion.

Illustration of catheter insertion, balloon inflation, and stent placement during cardiac catheterization

Cardiogenic Shock

The critical care nurse should be familiar with a dangerous condition known as **cardiogenic shock.** *Cardiogenic* means originating in the heart. **Shock** is a state in which blood flow in the body has dramatically decreased, and tissues are not getting adequate oxygen to perform their metabolic functions. Cardiogenic shock is when the heart has stopped pumping blood adequately through the body, characterized by critically low cardiac output, marked hypotension without volume loss, and signs of poor tissue perfusion such as cyanosis, oliguria, coolness of the extremities, and decreased level of consciousness. The nurse may see mottling of the skin in the legs and arms of the patient, detect a rapid and faint pulse, and auscultate distant-sounding heart sounds with a possible third and fourth heart sound present.

Cardiogenic shock often occurs following an acute MI. The ischemia that results from this condition causes the heart to fail in its ability to adequately circulate blood in the body. Mortality rates for cardiogenic shock are high if swift, aggressive intervention does not occur as soon as possible.

Cardiogenic shock is an emergency, and the patient must be treated immediately to prevent death. Admission to an ICU is likely, where the patient may have a central line put in to ensure rapid volume replacement and allow for multiple infusions of medicines to help maintain BP and cardiac output. The patient may have an arterial line placed to monitor BP continuously while BP is treated. Pharmacologic therapy will likely include drugs to improve cardiac contractility, such as dopamine, and diuretics to maintain volume and prevent volume overload during fluid resuscitation. If dopamine does not do an adequate job of maintaining BP, a stronger option would be norepinephrine, a potent vasoconstrictor. Any electrolyte abnormalities such as acidosis, hypokalemia, or hypomagnesemia will be corrected.

Some patients will have an intra-aortic balloon pump inserted in the aorta to assist the heart's function. When the heart pumps, during systole, the balloon is deflated. When the heart rests, during diastole, the balloon inflates. This inflation helps push blood into the coronary arteries, reperfusing them. The deflation allows for more space in the aorta and thus more blood to flow out to the body and the tissues needing oxygen.

Patients in cardiogenic shock are likely candidates for a percutaneous intervention (PCI) or coronary artery bypass graft (CABG) surgery to immediately correct the issue. Research has shown that a PCI is most effective within 90 minutes of patient presentation to prevent mortality and long-term damage.

Cardiomyopathies

A cardiomyopathy is any condition in which the heart muscle is diseased. There are four categories of cardiomyopathy that will be discussed here: dilated, hypertrophic, idiopathic, and restrictive cardiomyopathy.

Dilated

Dilated cardiomyopathy is a primary myocardial disorder, meaning it occurs on its own without any coronary artery disease or anything else. Usually both ventricles will be affected, and will be dilating, thinning, becoming hypertrophic, and causing systolic dysfunction. Mitral and tricuspid regurgitation often develop because of the dilation. When the left ventricle is affected, the patient will have exertional dyspnea and fatigue because the left ventricle diastolic pressure rises and cardiac output is reduced. When the right ventricle is affected, the patient may present with edema of the legs and arms along with jugular vein distention. The symptoms of dilated cardiomyopathy typically develop slowly over time, except for acute cases such as takotsubo.

Takotsubo cardiomyopathy, also known as **acute apical ballooning cardiomyopathy** or **broken heart syndrome**, is triggered by a sudden and extreme amount of emotional distress. The patient may have experienced the loss of a loved one or some other catastrophic life event, which set in motion a hyperadrenergic state in the body. *Takotsubo* is a Japanese word for a fishing pot used for capturing octopuses, which is what the left ventricle has been said to look like during this type of cardiomyopathy. Patients typically present in ways like those experiencing an ischemic event, with dyspnea, chest pain, nausea, and vomiting, among other symptoms. This type of heart failure is typically reversible, requiring acute hemodynamic support and similar treatment to patients with acute coronary syndrome.

Typical dilated cardiomyopathy has several different potential causes, including chronic tachycardia, connective tissue disorders such as rheumatoid arthritis, drugs and toxins such as alcohol and cocaine, inherited genetic factors, infections, and metabolic disorders such as diabetes mellitus. Viral infections are a well-known cause of dilated cardiomyopathy, with over twenty different viruses identified, such as human immunodeficiency virus (HIV) infection.

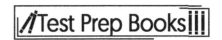

A patient with dilated cardiomyopathy will be diagnosed using a chest x-ray, which will show the enlargement of the heart, called **cardiomegaly**. The chest film may also show pleural effusions, a result of ventricular failure. Serological markers such as troponin may be elevated in dilated cardiomyopathy. Tissue samples from the heart muscle may be obtained for biopsy in some cases. ECG and imaging studies such as echocardiography and cardiac magnetic resonance imaging (MRI) will also be used to make a diagnosis of dilated cardiomyopathy.

Patients with dilated cardiomyopathy will be treated with angiotensin-converting enzyme (ACE) inhibitors, beta blockers, angiotensin-receptor blockers (ARBs), diuretics, and digoxin, among other pharmacologic therapies. These drugs are often used in heart failure with a lowered ejection fraction. **Ejection fraction** is a term of measurement used to quantify the percentage of blood leaving the heart with each beat. A patient with heart failure, as is the case with dilated cardiomyopathy, will have a much lower ejection fraction than normal. A normal ejection fraction is around 55 to 70 percent.

Hypertrophic
Hypertrophic cardiomyopathy is an inherited condition due to a genetic mutation. In very rare cases, this type of cardiomyopathy may be acquired, as is the case in patients with acromegaly. **Hypertrophy** refers to a thickening of the cardiac muscle, often becoming stiff and noncompliant. Ejection fraction in patients with hypertrophic cardiomyopathy may be elevated as the smaller heart chamber empties completely with each beat to maintain cardiac output.

This type of cardiomyopathy often occurs in athletes, frequently causing sudden death and the official diagnosis being made upon autopsy. Symptoms are like acute coronary artery occlusion, such as chest pain, dyspnea, and syncope. Patients will be diagnosed using echocardiography or cardiac MRI, where the heart structures are visualized and the severity of the hypertrophy is analyzed.

Family history of sudden death or patient history of unexplained syncope are clues that the patient may have this type of cardiomyopathy.

The treatment plan for a patient diagnosed with hypertrophic cardiomyopathy usually includes beta-blockers, such as metoprolol, and calcium channel blockers, such as verapamil. Beta-blockers and calcium channel blockers help with this type of cardiomyopathy because they slow the heart rate, decrease contractility, and prolong the time the heart chambers can fill between beats. Nitrates, diuretics, and ACE inhibitors should be avoided because they reduce preload, which worsens the condition. Implantable cardioverter defibrillator (ICD) is recommended to prevent death in patients with a history of cardiac arrest and syncope.

Idiopathic
When the cause of the cardiomyopathy is unknown, it is called **idiopathic**. This type of cardiomyopathy is responsible for up to half of the occurrences of heart failure. Patients with this type of cardiomyopathy are typically between twenty and sixty years of age. Their clinical presentation will be like other patients experiencing cardiomyopathy, with fatigue and dyspnea on exertion being a primary symptom if the left ventricle is affected. If the right ventricle is affected, jugular vein distention and edema may be present.

Like the other types of cardiomyopathies, idiopathic cardiomyopathy is believed to be the result of a viral infection, immune dysfunction, genetic factors, toxins, metabolism, and/or tachycardia-induced conditions. Alcohol and chemotherapeutic drugs are believed to be toxins that may cause cardiomyopathy.

The role of viruses must be investigated when determining the cause of idiopathic cardiomyopathy, as this root cause starts the chain reaction of inflammation and autoimmune dysfunction leading to cardiomyopathy. Viruses that have been associated with this type of cardiomyopathy include herpes, adenovirus, and enterovirus.

Treatment for the patient with idiopathic cardiomyopathy may include lifestyle modification of risk factors such as alcohol abuse; drug therapy with ACE inhibitors, beta-blockers, diuretics, and digitalis; and possible resynchronization therapy in patients experiencing dysrhythmias. Patients experiencing cardiomyopathy in the absence of a viral cause may be good candidates for immunosuppressive therapies such as prednisone, per the discretion of the physician.

Restrictive

A cardiomyopathy characterized by noncompliant heart walls that are resistant to filling during the diastolic period is termed **restrictive cardiomyopathy**. There are two categories of restrictive cardiomyopathy: obliterative and nonobliterative. **Obliterative** means that there is fibrosis within the endocardium and subendocardium, while **nonobliterative** entails that the myocardium has been infiltrated by an abnormal substance. One or both ventricles of the heart may be affected. Restrictive cardiomyopathy is much less common than dilated, idiopathic, and hypertrophic cardiomyopathies.

A patient with restrictive cardiomyopathy may present with fatigue and exertional dyspnea, like the other cardiomyopathic presentations. This is due to decreased cardiac output and oxygen delivery to the tissues and organs of the body.

Restrictive cardiomyopathy may arise because of genetic factors. The resistance to diastolic filling results in an increased filling pressure, followed by pulmonary venous hypertension.

A patient will be diagnosed with restrictive cardiomyopathy using echocardiography to visualize the ventricles and other structures of the heart. Cardiac MRI, heart catheterization, and biopsy may also be used to confirm the diagnosis.

A patient diagnosed with restrictive cardiomyopathy has a poor prognosis, unfortunately, as diagnosis is often made in the later stages of the disease. The cause will be treated if possible along with supportive treatment for symptoms. Diuretics will be used to relieve pulmonary vascular congestion if appropriate.

Illustration comparing a normal heart muscle with dilated, hypertrophic, and restrictive cardiomyopathies

| Normal | Dilated | Hypertrophic | Restrictive |

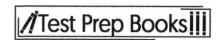

Dysrhythmias

A normal, healthy heart is a muscular pump powered by an electrical current that passes throughout its myocytes with every beat. The electrical impulse that triggers heart contractions can be measured using an ECG. In a disease state, abnormalities in electrical activity and conduction arise leading to irregular contractions of the chambers of the heart, called **dysrhythmias**.

Normal or sinus rhythm involves regular contraction of the atria followed by contraction of the ventricles. Atrial contraction fills the ventricles, and ventricle contraction pushes the blood to the lungs to be oxygenated or to the body to distribute the blood. Normal heart rate in an adult is 60 to 100 beats per minute. Slower rates are called **bradycardia,** while faster rates are called **tachycardia**.

A **fibrillation** is a movement of the heart best described as a flutter or a quiver. It is an ineffectual contraction of a chamber of the heart, in which inadequate blood flow is produced. Atrial fibrillation, often shortened to "AFib," is an abnormal but constant and rapid rhythm of the atria. A fib puts the patient at risk for the formation of clots in the atrial chambers. These clots, formed in pooling blood that is not adequately pumped out of the heart, may dislodge and travel to other parts of the body, such as the heart and brain, causing ischemic syndromes.

While a patient can live with AFib for some time without knowing it or needing much treatment, ventricular fibrillation is a different story. When the ventricles fibrillate and fail to adequately pump blood out of the body, it is a medical emergency requiring immediate intervention. Cardiopulmonary resuscitation with defibrillation is necessary, the pumping action of chest compressions making up for the ventricular failure in perfusing vital organs. Ventricular failure is the presenting rhythm for most patients experiencing cardiac arrest, often being the ultimate cause of death if resuscitation is unsuccessful.

Other common heart dysrhythmias include atrial flutter, atrioventricular block, bundle branch block (BBB), long QT syndrome, torsades de pointes, and ventricular tachycardia.

Heart Failure

In a normal heart, when preload increases, the heart rises to meet the demand, pumping harder and faster to maintain perfusion of vital body organs. In heart failure, the heart no longer is able to meet the demands of the body, with weakened contractions and less cardiac output.

The Frank-Starling Law of the Heart describes the relationship between preload, heart contractility, and heart failure. In heart failure, the heart can no longer meet the demands of preload, and decreased contractility and cardiac output result.

Heart failure can arise from many different causes, including myocardial damage from an MI, disorders of the heart valves such as aortic stenosis, arrhythmias (both bradycardia and tachycardia), defects in the conduction system such as a left BBB, or even systemic disorders such as anemia, hyperthyroidism, and hypertension.

Treatment is available and can help with overall quality of life, but no cure is currently available. Drug therapy will target symptoms with diuretics, nitrates, or digoxin with long-term management in the form of ACE inhibitors, beta-blockers, and ARBs. Some patients may have an ICD placed to help with dysrhythmias and to resuscitate them should they go into cardiac arrest. Surgeries such as valve repairs, CABG, and even heart transplantation may be considered.

Hypertensive Crisis

A patient may present to the urgent care center or emergency room with an uncontrollably high BP, with a systolic reading greater than 200 and a diastolic reading greater than 120. BP this high, rightly-called **malignant hypertension**, can cause damage to the organs supplied by the blood vessels, such as the heart, kidneys, brain, and lungs. A hypertensive crisis may arise if the patient forgets to take their BP medication, they've experienced a heart attack or stroke, their kidneys are failing, and many other scenarios.

Symptoms of high BP include a severe headache, severe chest pain, nausea and vomiting, anxiety, shortness of breath, seizures, and unresponsiveness.

Upon presentation with malignant hypertension, the doctor may decide to infuse intravenous (IV) medications to reduce the BP. Such medications include sodium nitroprusside and esmolol, a beta-blocker. The clinician will be very careful not to lower the BP too quickly, as a dramatic drop in BP could cause further damage to end organs.

Possible comorbidities of a hypertensive crisis include the organs that such a high BP could damage: cerebral vascular accident, myocardial ischemia or infarction, bleeding in the brain such as subarachnoid hemorrhage, pulmonary edema, aortic dissection, and acute renal failure.

Extremely high BP in pregnancy is called **preeclampsia** or **eclampsia**. Women experiencing this condition may be given hydralazine to lower their pressure, which presents not only a danger to them but to the forming fetus in the uterus. Magnesium sulfate is also given to pregnant women to prevent them from experiencing a seizure while hypertensive.

Myocardial Conduction System Defects

Myocardial conduction refers to the movement of an electrical impulse across the myocytes, or muscle cells, that causes contractions. Common conduction disorders include bundle branch blocks (BBBs), heart block, and long QT syndrome.

BBBs occur when there is a block in either the right, left, or both branches of the heart's conduction system, traveling the length of the ventricles. A patient with BBB may be asymptomatic, as the heart compensates by having the electrical impulse travel down a different path than the blocked branch to stimulate ventricular contraction. The ventricle affected will then beat just a fraction of a second slower than the other one, not producing any noticeable symptoms. BBB will likely be found when diagnosing some other heart condition, but it is good to know it is there. No treatment is usually required if the patient is asymptomatic.

A **heart block** is any instance in which the electrical impulse of the heart does not travel correctly from the atria to the ventricles, occurring in varying degrees from first degree to third degree. First-degree heart blocks are defined by a slower movement of the electrical signal, while second-degree heart blocks are defined by missed beats caused by electrical impulses that never reach the ventricles. In third-degree, or complete heart block, the electrical impulse is not passing to the lower chambers at all, resulting in ineffective blood pumping and a very slow heart rate. Patients with third-degree heart block will likely need a pacemaker implanted.

Long QT syndrome occurs when the QT segment of the ECG wave form is prolonged, representing the electrical activity in the ventricles. This hereditary and rare disorder usually occurs in healthy adults and

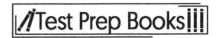

children and is characterized by fainting episodes, feelings of "fluttering" in the chest, and abnormal heart rate or rhythm. Diagnosis occurs with ECG and stress testing. Long QT syndrome may be fatal, as it could potentially cause sudden cardiac arrest. A treatment plan for long QT syndrome may include beta-blockers, avoiding drugs that aggravate the syndrome, and possibly implantation of an ICD or pacemaker.

Structural Heart Defects

The most common types of heart defects occur in developing fetuses and are diagnosed shortly after the child is born. Some common types of congenital defects are atrial septal defects (ASDs), patent foramen ovale (PFO), patent ductus arteriosus, coarctation of the aorta, and tetralogy of Fallot.

ASD and PFO are similar in that there is a hole between the two atria of the heart, and oxygen-rich blood leaks from the left chamber to the right. In ASD, the tissue never forms, and in PFO, the hole that is normally there does not close after birth as it should. An ASD hole is generally larger than a PFO.

Patent ductus arteriosus occurs when the **ductus arteriosus**, the vessel that connects the pulmonary artery and the aorta, does not close as it should after birth. The ductus arteriosus is vital for fetal development, but if it remains open after birth, the oxygen-rich blood of the aorta that is meant for body circulation gets mixed with the oxygen-poor blood of the pulmonary artery, resulting in increased pulmonary pressures and stress on the heart.

A narrowing of the aorta in a baby is called **coarctation of the aorta** and results in hypertension and heart damage.

Tetralogy of Fallot is a complex congenital heart defect involving four defects: a hole between the two ventricles called a **ventricular septal defect (VSD)**, pulmonary valve stenosis, an aorta that is located between the two ventricles and above the VSD, and hypertrophy, or a thickening of the right ventricle due to working harder because of the pulmonary valve stenosis. Patients with tetralogy of Fallot must have open heart surgery to repair the defects.

Structural Heart Defects

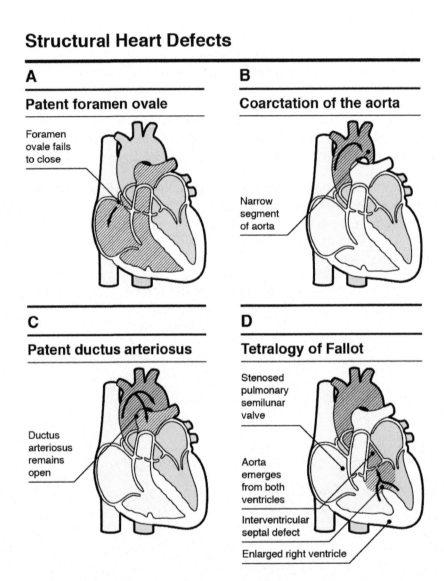

A

Patent foramen ovale

Foramen ovale fails to close

B

Coarctation of the aorta

Narrow segment of aorta

C

Patent ductus arteriosus

Ductus arteriosus remains open

D

Tetralogy of Fallot

Stenosed pulmonary semilunar valve

Aorta emerges from both ventricles

Interventricular septal defect

Enlarged right ventricle

Structural heart defects occurring in adulthood include valvular disease. There are four valves in the heart: mitral, tricuspid, aortic, and pulmonary. These valves control the flow of blood between the chambers of the heart as well as the lungs for oxygenation and the body for circulation. Valvular defects occur because of normal aging and degeneration, infections, high BP, atherosclerosis, ischemic conditions such as heart attack, tumors, radiation, and even some medications. Valve dysfunctions can include stiffening, in which blood is forced backward rather than forward, or weakening, in which blood leaks inappropriately between chambers. The severity of the valve dysfunction determines the number of symptoms and the amount and type of treatment needed. Patients with valvular disease may experience palpitations, fatigue, dizziness, and/or chest pain. Diagnosis is made with an ECG, stress tests, chest x-rays, echocardiograms, and/or cardiac catheterization. Smoking cessation will be

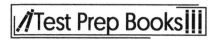

encouraged, antithrombotics or anticoagulants may be used to prevent dangerous clotting, and surgery to repair the valves may be a possibility for the patient with valvular disease.

Ruptured or Dissecting Aneurysms

A patient experiencing a sudden onset of tearing chest pain may be experiencing a rupture or dissection of an aortic aneurysm. Aortic aneurysms may occur at the top of the aorta, right after exiting the heart, termed **thoracic aortic aneurysms**. Aortic aneurysms may also occur farther down the aorta, then called either **thoracoabdominal aortic aneurysms** or **abdominal aortic aneurysms**. An **aneurysm** is any ballooning or enlargement of a blood vessel, often caused by atherosclerosis. When an aneurysm suddenly tears apart, massive amounts of the patient's blood start surging out with each and every heartbeat, making it an immediate medical emergency. A patient experiencing an aortic aneurysm dissection needs immediate surgical repair followed by intense cardiac and hemodynamic monitoring until stabilized.

Patients with unruptured aortic aneurysms may be completely asymptomatic. Detection of an aortic aneurysm occurs through ultrasonography, abdominal CT, echocardiography, and/or transesophageal echocardiography. Treatment for aortic aneurysms that have not ruptured includes elective surgical repair along with encouragement to quit smoking, a major cause of atherosclerosis, and drug therapy including antilipids and BP control.

Illustration showing the difference between an abdominal and thoracic aortic aneurysm

A

An abdominothoracic aneurysm spans the length above and below the kidneys.

Aorta exiting heart

Heart

Artery to kidneys

Kidneys

B

Thoracic aorta

Thoracic aortic aneurysm

C

Abdominal aorta

Abdominal aortic aneurysm

19/27 = 70.37%

Practice Questions

1. A STEMI, in which the full thickness of the heart wall has been damaged, results in which of the following ECG changes? *full thickness damage*
   a. T-wave inversion *= NSTEMI*
   b. ST-segment elevation
   c. QT prolongation *= irregular, chaotic rhythms, Ø MI*
   d. U-wave elevation *= hypokalemia*

2. What is one way a woman may present differently than a man when experiencing a heart attack?
   a. Symptoms beginning days to weeks before actual attack
   b. Profuse sweating *classic in men/women*
   c. Crushing chest pain
   d. Elevated serological markers
   woman symptoms = flulike, anxiety, jaw/back pain

3. What other condition may mimic the symptoms of a heart attack?
   a. Cirrhosis of the liver
   b. Kidney failure
   c. Acid reflux → *also anxiety/panic attacks*
   d. Pneumonia

X 4. What serological marker indicates, with high specificity, that cardiac muscle tissue has been damaged and cell contents are being released into the bloodstream?
   a. Creatinine *= renal failure*
   b. BUN
   c. Creatine kinase *X = similar to skeletal muscle, cardic enzyme less specific but*
   d. Troponin *muscle cell protein released when cardiac tissue breaks down w/ ischemia*
   cardiac exclusive enzyme

5. Which of the following statements about the cardiac catheterization procedure is true?
   a. The brachial artery is a common access site. *Ø fem A*
   b. The thin tube threaded into the patient's heart has a camera called a scope on the end for visualization of heart structures. *Ø camera or scope*
   c. Angioplasty and stent placement are commonly performed to open occluded coronary vessels. *dye shot under fluoro*
   d. The patient is put under general anesthesia for the procedure. *Ø conc sedation*

6. What type of rupture of muscles anchoring the atrioventricular valves can follow an ischemic event such as a myocardial infarction and lead to patient death if left untreated?
   a. Pupillary *= eye*
   b. Papillary *that anchor AV valves (mitral/tricuspid)*
   c. Pectoralis
   d. Palmaris *= hand*
   MI ↓ rupture caused = regurg/pulm edema, cardiogenic shock, death

X 7. Over what area of the heart will the nurse auscultate a holosystolic murmur accompanied by a thrill when there is a mitral regurgitation caused by papillary muscle rupture following an MI?
   a. Aortic
   b. Tricuspid
   c. Pulmonic
   d. Apical
   aortic systolic
   Pulmonic → systolic ejection murmur (flow/pulm stenosis)
   Tricuspid = Tricuspid → ASD (diastolic), tricuspid stenosis (diastolic), tricuspid regurg
   Apical = mitral
   ↳ mitral regurg, stenosis, valve prolapse
   holosystolic ↑ diastolic systolic ↑ or VSD cholosys

8. Which of the following would NOT indicate arterial insufficiency?
   a. Cyanosis of lower extremities
   b. Loss of hair in legs
   c. Sores that will not heal
   d. Pooling of blood and edema

arteries bring O2
= venous insufficiency rather than arterial

9. What is the most common cause of edema caused by venous insufficiency?
   a. Deep vein thrombosis (DVT) *most common cause*
   b. Obesity X
   c. Pregnancy
   d. Old age
   relative / potential

10. What test is often used to determine if a patient has peripheral arterial disease?
   a. Echocardiography *= sonography visualizing structures of ♡*
   b. CT scan of the leg *= Ø useful*
   c. Electrocardiogram *= electrical conduction*
   d. Ankle-brachial BP index *"ABIs" = flow → compares blood pressure in 2 sites (assess flow)*

11. For an episode of neurological deficits to be considered a transient ischemic attack (TIA) versus a cerebrovascular accident (CVA), what is the time frame?
   a. More than 1 hour but less than 2 hours
   b. More than 5 minutes but less than 1 hour *, if symptoms > 1H will likely cause/result in CVA ischemic ↗*
   c. More than 45 minutes but less than 1 hour
   d. More than 2 hours but less than 3 hours

12. What risk does high blood pressure pose in the postoperative period following an endarterectomy?
   a. Bleeding *= low blood pressure sign*
   b. Infection X
   c. Pulmonary edema X
   d. Stroke

13. What type of drug therapy coupled with antithrombotic therapy is often used post-endarterectomy?
   a. Antiplatelet *= ↓ stickiness of blood*
   b. Beta-blocker
   c. Angiotensin-converting enzyme
   d. Angiotensin II receptor blockers

14. What is the main concern faced when using an artificial graft to bypass an occluded artery in the fem-pop bypass procedure?
   a. Localized infection
   b. Narrowing leading to reocclusion *fem/popliteal, known complications*
   c. Lower extremity edema
   d. Tissue rejection X

15. Which type of drug class is often used to reduce preload in cardiogenic pulmonary edema?
   a. Beta-blockers such as metoprolol *slow HR*
   b. Calcium channel blockers such as verapamil *for dysrhythmias*
   c. Narcotics such as morphine *↓ air hunger / ↓ anxiety*
   d. Diuretics such as furosemide

33

16. Which of the following is NOT a toxic effect of nicotine inhaled during cigarette smoking?
    a. Plaque buildup = atherosclerosis ø specific nicotine inhal
    b. Inflammation of endothelium
    c. Vasoconstriction of blood vessels   toxic effects of smoking
    d. Hypertension

17. What differentiating factor would let a nurse know that a lower extremity ulcer is arterial rather than venous?
    a. Color of wound
    b. Culture taken from wound infection
    c. Depth of wound arterial ulcer = nonhealing/deep, exposing tendons/bone
    d. Measurement of wound irrelevant

18. Which of the following is NOT a usual sign that a patient is in shock?
    a. Increased urine output normally oliguric
    b. Distant heart sounds
    c. Bluish tinted skin   normal shock state
    d. Faint and rapid pulse

19. If dopamine does not do an adequate job of maintaining blood pressure in a patient experiencing cardiogenic shock, which potent vasoconstrictor will be considered to raise the blood pressure?
    a. Dobutamine stronger beta effects, used for dilation
    b. Norepinephrine potent vasoconstrictor
    c. Milrinone vaso dilation/⊕ inotrope
    d. Nitroglycerin vasodilator, ↓BP

20. The balloon pump inflates during diastole for what purpose in a patient experiencing cardiogenic shock?
    a. To allow more space in the aorta deflation stage
    b. To push more blood flow out into the peripheral circulation deflation stage
    c. To raise blood pressure in hypotensive states ↑ HF
    d. To encourage perfusion of coronary arteries and diastolic filling of the heart ↑CO w/ afterload reduction

21. Which item in the family history assessment performed by the critical care nurse is a red flag for hypertrophic cardiomyopathy and should be investigated further?
    a. Heart disease of the father X ø
    b. Diabetes mellitus of the mother ø
    c. Sudden death of a grandmother couldve been dx before, pt often asymptomatic
    d. Stroke of a grandfather ø   + syncope/sudden death occurs

22. What is the most common and deadly heart rhythm detected in patients experiencing cardiac arrest?
    a. Atrial fibrillation
    b. Ventricular tachycardia
    c. Ventricular fibrillation most common, uncondus/unrespnsive
    d. Supraventricular tachycardia

34

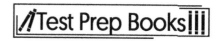

23. According to the Frank-Starling law of the heart, a patient with heart failure will respond to an increase in preload in which of the following ways?
    a. Increased contractility
    b. Decreased cardiac output
    c. Change in rhythm
    d. Increased heart rate

Handwritten: HR x SV = CO ; HF Ø respond to extra preload, ↓CO ; p↑ in

24. An 8-month-pregnant woman presents to the ED with eclampsia. Which IV medication will be given to prevent seizures?
    a. Magnesium sulfate
    b. Sodium chloride
    c. Dextrose in water
    d. Potassium supplement

Handwritten: = prevent SZ ; Ø specific to pregnancy

25. What myocardial conduction defect is hereditary, may result in syncope or sudden death, and often occurs in healthy adults or children?
    a. Third-degree heart block
    b. First-degree heart block
    c. Bundle branch block
    d. Long QT syndrome

Handwritten: = miscommunication between atria/ventricles ; = interruption between ventricles ; = rare, hereditary condition, healthy children/adults asymptomatic until syncopal episode/sudden death

26. Which of the following is not a congenital heart defect found in the tetralogy of Fallot?
    a. Pulmonary valve stenosis
    b. Ventricular septal defect
    c. Atrial septal defect
    d. Hypertrophic right ventricle

Handwritten: tetralogy of Fallot ; tetralogy of Fallot present @ birth ; ① VSD ② aorta from both ventricles ③ hypertrophic RV ④ pulm valve stenosis

27. Which of the following lifestyle modifications would address the major cause of most aortic aneurysms?
    a. Low-fat diet
    b. Smoking cessation
    c. Exercise program
    d. Meditation

Handwritten: contributing factor ; major cause of atherosclerosis, most common cause

Answer Explanations

1. B: An ST-segment elevation is the classic ECG reading that indicates a STEMI, in which the full thickness of the heart wall has been damaged, leading to the significant ECG changes. T-wave inversion can be linked to a number of cardiac disorders, both benign and life-threatening, but in the case of heart attacks, it is linked to NSTEMIs. The QT-segment prolongation is part of a condition in which the patient experiences irregular, chaotic heart rhythms from time to time and is not associated with an active myocardial infarction. The U wave is sometimes too small to be observed on a normal ECG. It follows the T wave and is not significant in showing heart wall damage, although it can become elevated in hypokalemia.

2. A: A woman may have flulike symptoms, anxiety, or jaw or back pain days to weeks before the actual cardiac event. These symptoms may be overlooked and the correct diagnosis missed if the clinician is unaware of gender differences. The other three choices listed are classic, well-known symptoms of a myocardial infarction in both men and women.

3. C: Acid reflux, along with anxiety or panic attacks, may mimic the chest pain experienced during a heart attack. The proximity of the upper sphincters of the stomach involved in acid reflux to the heart muscle are the cause of the confusion. The patient's presentation, history, and physical along with lab testing and assessment will aid in correct diagnosis. While liver cirrhosis, kidney failure, and pneumonia all involve organs close to the heart, they do not mimic the symptoms of a heart attack.

4. D: Troponin is a muscle cell protein that is released when cardiac tissue is broken down during an ischemic event. Elevated levels of troponin in the bloodstream indicate cardiac muscle damage. Creatinine and BUN are waste products of the body, and higher levels of these in the bloodstream indicate kidney failure or damage, not heart damage. Creatine kinase is an enzyme found in muscle tissue. One form of the enzyme, CK-MB, is a cardiac enzyme, but its structure is similar to creatine kinase found in skeletal muscle. Therefore, it's a less specific indicator of cardiac muscle damage.

5. C: Angioplasty and stent placement often occur during routine cardiac catheterization to open up occluded blood vessels. There is no camera or scope; instead, dye is shot through the catheter and x-ray images are obtained to visualize structures. The femoral artery is the most commonly accessed blood vessel for left heart catheterization versus the brachial artery, which can be used but is not as common. The patient is not put to sleep, but rather given medicine to help them relax while keeping them awake.

6. B: The five papillary muscles located in the heart anchor the atrioventricular valves—the mitral and tricuspid, to be specific. When these muscles fall apart and rupture after an ischemic event such as a myocardial infarction, the valves begin to regurgitate, causing pulmonary edema followed by cardiogenic shock and ultimately death if left untreated. *Pupillary* refers to the eye. *Pectoralis* and *palmaris* refer to the pectoral and palm muscles of the body and are thus unrelated.

7. D: An apical holosystolic murmur accompanied by a thrill may be noted when a patient has experienced papillary muscle rupture following an MI. The aortic, tricuspid, and pulmonic auscultation points will not bring out the same auscultated sounds, as they are not as close to the mitral valve that has been affected by the event.

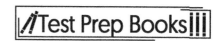

8. D: The pooling of blood and edematous swelling are signs of a venous insufficiency rather than an arterial one. Remember, arteries bring oxygen, so when there is a lack of oxygen, tissue cannot get oxygen, thus causing cyanosis and hair loss, and sores or wounds cannot heal. When venous blood is not returning to the heart, pooling and edema occur.

9. A: DVT is the most common cause of edema caused by venous insufficiency. The other three factors are also potential causes, but are not as common as DVT.

10. D: An ankle-brachial BP index is commonly used to diagnose peripheral arterial disease by comparing the blood pressures of the two sites, thus assessing blood flow. An echocardiogram is a sonographic test used to visualize the structures of the heart, such as in heart failure. A computed tomography (CT) scan would not be useful for visualizing arterial structures of the extremities, or at least it is not commonly used. An electrocardiogram is used to measure and track electrical activity of heart muscle.

11. B: For a neurologic attack to be considered transient, as in a transient ischemic attack (TIA), the stroke-like symptoms must last longer than 5 minutes but less than 1 hour. Greater than an hour will likely result in and/or indicate a cerebrovascular accident, in which brain tissue is damaged due to an ischemic event. The other three answers do not fall in line with this parameter.

12. D: A stroke is a potential complication of hypertension in a patient post-endarterectomy. The critical care nurse must carefully monitor and treat high blood pressure should it occur. Bleeding would be marked by low blood pressure. Infection is a noncardiac issue; thus, it is unrelated to blood pressure in this instance. Pulmonary edema can occur as a result of heart failure and is not pertinent to the monitoring for high blood pressure.

13. A: Antiplatelet therapy, commonly aspirin, is coupled with antithrombotic therapy in the postoperative period following endarterectomy to prevent clotting of blood caused by platelet aggregation, which would reocclude the blood vessels just operated on. Beta-blockers, ACE inhibitors, and ARBs are not commonly paired with antithrombotics; rather, they target blood pressure issues and heart failure.

14. B: When using an artificial graft, rather than a patient's own vessel, to graft in between the femoral and popliteal arteries in the leg, narrowing and reocclusion are a concern. This is a known complication of these types of grafts. Infection is always a risk but nonspecific to this instance. Edema is associated with venous occlusion and insufficiency. Tissue graft rejection is a possibility but was not mentioned specifically in the text.

15. D: Diuretics such as furosemide (Lasix®) will help reduce preload in a patient experiencing cardiogenic pulmonary edema. Metoprolol and other beta-blockers are used in heart failure to slow the beating of the heart. Calcium channel blockers, such as verapamil, are used for heart dysrhythmias such as atrial fibrillation and in some cases of heart failure, improving the heart's ability to pump. Narcotics such as morphine are sometimes used to reduce anxiety and oxygen hunger in acute cases of pulmonary edema.

16. A: Plaque buildup is a mark of atherosclerosis and is nonspecific to nicotine inhalation. The other three items listed—inflammation of the vascular endothelium, vasoconstriction, and increased blood pressure—are all effects of the toxic nature of nicotine inhalation due to cigarette smoking.

17. C: The depth of the wound is the biggest clue as to whether the ulcer arose out of an arterial insufficiency or a venous insufficiency. Arterial ulcers are usually nonhealing and deep, eventually exposing tendons and bones if left untreated. The color of the ulcer may vary across a spectrum, regardless of the type. Cultures from the wound only tell what types of infectious agents have entered the ulcerative tissue. The size or depth of the wound is irrelevant.

18. A: A patient in shock will usually exhibit oliguria, in which urine output has dramatically decreased or stopped altogether, signaling a shutting down of the kidneys due to lack of perfusion from the heart. Other signs of decreased perfusion as seen in a shock state are distant heart sounds, cyanosis, and faint and rapid pulse.

19. B: Norepinephrine is a potent vasoconstrictor that may be used if dobutamine is inadequate in maintaining normal blood pressure in a patient experiencing cardiogenic shock. Dobutamine is an option but is used for systemic vasodilation with stronger beta effects than the others mentioned here. Milrinone causes vasodilation and positive inotropic effects. Nitroglycerin is a potent vasodilator that would lower blood pressure rather than raise it.

20. D: When the balloon inflates during diastole, blood flow back into the coronary arteries and diastolic filling are encouraged, both which improve heart function. The first two options listed, creating space in the aorta and pushing more blood out into peripheral circulation, are effects of the deflation stage of the balloon pump's actions. The function of the balloon pump is not specifically aimed at raising blood pressure, though this may be an effect of improved heart function because of the pump.

21. C: The sudden death of a grandmother needs to be probed for if a cause was determined. If she passed away suddenly because of hypertrophic cardiomyopathy that had been previously undiagnosed before autopsy, the patient should be screened for this condition as well, as it often may be asymptomatic until syncope or sudden death occurs. The other three items listed are of value, but do not point toward hypertrophic cardiomyopathy specifically.

22. C: Ventricular fibrillation is the most common rhythm detected when a patient goes into cardiac arrest. This is because the fibrillation of the ventricles produces inadequate heart contraction to pump the blood to the vital organs. Without oxygen, the patient "falls out," becoming unconscious and unresponsive. Patients in ventricular fibrillation need immediate cardiopulmonary resuscitation—most importantly, defibrillation. The other rhythms mentioned—atrial fibrillation, ventricular tachycardia, and supraventricular tachycardia—may present serious complications for the patient and must be treated, but are not the most common cause of cardiac arrest.

23. B: A patient with heart failure will not be able to respond to increased preload as a normal, healthy patient would, resulting in decreased cardiac output. Contractility is not increased as well as in a healthy heart. Changes in rhythm and rate are not significant as far as patients with heart failure and their response to preload.

24. A: IV magnesium sulfate will be given to the pregnant woman experiencing eclampsia to prevent seizures. The other three IV medications listed are all used to correct fluid and electrolyte imbalances and may be used, but not specifically for the purpose of preventing seizures in a pregnant woman in hypertensive crisis.

25. D: Long QT syndrome is a rare, hereditary condition found many times in healthy children and adults that may be asymptomatic until a syncopal episode or even sudden death occurs. First- and third-degree heart block occurs when there are conduction problems between the atria and ventricles, resulting in "missed" heartbeats. Bundle branch block occurs when there is an interruption in the electrical impulse across the ventricles of the heart.

26. C: An atrial septal defect is not part of the tetralogy of Fallot. The tetralogy of Fallot includes a ventricular septal defect, an aorta arising from both ventricles, and hypertrophy of the overworked right ventricle due to pulmonary valve stenosis.

27. B: Cigarette smoking is a major cause of atherosclerosis, the most common cause of aortic aneurysm. Following a low-fat diet would help with dyslipidemia, which may be a contributor to atherosclerosis, but not as important as smoking cessation, which causes the inflammatory, toxic effects that produce atherosclerosis. Exercise is helpful in coping with stress effectively, as is meditation, but not specific to atherosclerosis that causes aortic aneurysms.

Pulmonary

Working in tandem with the cardiac system is the pulmonary system, composed of the two lungs and the airway. Airway and breathing are part of the airway, breathing, circulation (ABC) mnemonic representing the patient's most vital functions. The critical care nurse knows that taking good care of the patient's pulmonary system using critical thinking and sound clinical judgments is crucial to the patient's overall well-being.

The following is a discussion of the major critical care situations involving the pulmonary system, patient presentation, and course of treatment.

Acute Pulmonary Embolus

One potential complication for a patient in a critical care unit is a PE. A PE is a clot that has developed elsewhere in the body, traveled to the pulmonary arteries, and occluded at least one, if not more, of them. PEs often develop in the deep, large, femoral or pelvic veins of the body, become dislodged, and travel up through the right side of the heart, through the pulmonary artery, and into the lungs.

There are three categories of PEs based on severity: small, submassive, and massive. Small PEs may exist without any symptoms. Submassive PEs may slightly impair right ventricular function, but hypotension is absent. A massive PE impairs the function of the right ventricle, causes a hypotensive crisis, and presents a serious risk of death for the patient.

A saddle PE is a particularly dangerous type of clot in which the pulmonary embolus has lodged itself in the bifurcation between the main pulmonary artery and the left and right pulmonary arteries. Saddle PEs usually impair right ventricular function with or without hypotension.

Detection of PEs is somewhat difficult. Practitioners may use a D-Dimer test to rule out or indicate the probability of a PE. V/Q scans, in which ventilation and perfusion of the lungs is evaluated, may assist in diagnosis. CT scanning is the best way to image a PE, although patients with renal failure will not be able to tolerate the contrast, and thus, V/Q scanning is used.

Treatment of a PE includes reducing the clot burden in the patient through anticoagulants such as IV heparin, subcutaneous fondaparinux, and/or IV argatroban. Any patient on anticoagulant therapy is at risk for bleeding and should be monitored for such.

Warfarin may be used for long-term anticoagulation therapy in patients at risk for clotting but should be checked for interactions with other medications. Patients on warfarin will also have to have their international normalized ratio (INR) checked periodically to monitor the effectiveness of anticoagulation.

Prevention is key with PEs. Patients who remain immobile and in bed are at risk for developing clots. These clots may start as DVTs and then travel to the lungs to create PEs, a life-threatening event in many patients. Early anticoagulation when PEs or DVTs are possible along with early patient mobilization are key to prevention.

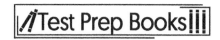

Acute Respiratory Distress Syndrome (ARDS)

When a patient is in respiratory failure that is unresponsive to supplemental oxygen with marked hypoxemia, it is called **acute respiratory distress syndrome (ARDS)** or sometimes **acute hypoxemic respiratory failure (AHRF)**. This type of respiratory failure may be caused by acute lung injury (ALI) and can occur in the conditions that predispose a patient to any sort of respiratory distress syndrome (RDS).

When the blood is not adequately oxygenated because of poor oxygen exchange in the alveoli in the lungs, the patient will become dyspneic, and oxygen saturation readings will drop. A pulse oxygenation of below 90 percent is considered below normal in most patients and must be treated. If the patient is not responding to inhaled oxygen therapy through nasal prongs or even high flows of 70 to 100 percent oxygen on a nonrebreather face mask, mechanical ventilation will be the next step in treating ARDS.

Mechanical ventilation can assist in ARDS by relieving the work of the heart and respiratory muscles, distributing cardiac output to other vital tissues in the body while the vent takes over the work of breathing. By maintaining a positive end-expiratory pressure (PEEP), the vent can stave off pulmonary edema, recruiting more alveoli to participate in oxygen exchange.

A patient with ARDS will be diagnosed beginning with pulse oxygenation. When the blood oxygen concentration drops below 90, causes will be investigated, ARDS will be considered, chest x-ray obtained, and arterial blood glasses (ABGs) taken. The chest x-ray may show infiltrates indicating pulmonary edema and/or pneumonia, which are other possible causes of ARDS. The ABGs will indicate oxygenation as well as any acidotic or alkalotic states of the blood. A mild amount of acidosis may be tolerated in the patient when the greater good of ventilation and oxygenation are being maintained. An acidotic pH of less than 7.15, however, may be treated with IV sodium bicarbonate.

ALI can arise from direct and indirect causes. A direct cause would be gastric acid aspiration or pneumonia. Indirect causes of lung injury include sepsis or trauma arising from prolonged hypovolemic shock.

Propofol is a preferred sedative for patients on mechanical ventilation, as breathing with the vent is highly uncomfortable. The patient may become agitated and "fight the vent," causing uncoordinated breaths and further problems with oxygenation and ventilation. Other analgesics that may be considered are fentanyl and morphine.

Acute Respiratory Failure

Any case in which oxygen exchange in the alveoli of the lungs is impaired, whether due to impaired respiration, weakness of respiratory effort, or obstruction of the airway, is called **respiratory failure**. Though respiratory arrest and cardiac arrest are two different events, one always leads to another if one is left untreated. Lack of oxygen will cause permanent damage to vital organs if respiratory arrest goes on for much longer than five minutes.

Respiratory failure can occur because of an upper or lower airway obstruction. Upper airway obstructions include blood, mucus, foreign object, tumor, inflammation, or edema. Lower airway obstructions include aspiration, bronchospasm, pneumonia, pulmonary edema or hemorrhage, or drowning.

Patients with central nervous system deficits may have a decreased respiratory effort, leading to respiratory failure. Examples of this include brain stem injuries as is the case with strokes and tumors.

An adverse medication effect may cause decreased respiratory effort. Alcohol, opioids, and sedatives are all examples of drugs that can depress respiratory effort to the point of failure.

Hypoglycemia and hypotension are examples of metabolic disorders that may weaken respiratory effort.

The critical care nurse will recognize a patient going into respiratory distress by observing lowered respiratory effort, difficulty breathing, unconsciousness, cyanosis, and lowered pulse oxygenation percentages. Patients that may be on the cusp of a respiratory arrest may exhibit signs of decreasing neurologic function such as agitation, confusion, and oxygen hunger. They may be sweating profusely and have a rapid heart rate.

Diagnosis of respiratory failure will be based off clinical observation, and treatment will depend on the cause. If there is an obstruction present, it will need to be removed. If failure was caused by an adverse drug effect, an antidote may be given if appropriate. More than likely, the patient in respiratory failure will be aggressively ventilated using mechanical ventilation if necessary to prevent impending cardiac arrest. Oxygenation and ventilation are the high priority at this point.

Acute Respiratory Infections

One of the most common and deadly lung infections a patient can succumb to is pneumonia. Pneumonia is an inflammation of the lung tissue caused by some sort of infection, whether bacterial, viral, fungal, or parasitic. Most pneumonias are bacterial, usually *Streptococcus pneumoniae.*

Everyone breathes in pathogens daily. The upper airways are colonized with "normal" flora. The difference is when a patient becomes immunocompromised or a particularly virulent pathogen is introduced. The normal responses of mucociliary clearance, cough, and the actions of the white blood cells are no longer effective, and infection results.

There are five categories of pneumonia based on how and where the pneumonia is acquired: community, hospital, health care associated, immunocompromised, and aspiration. Aspiration pneumonia will be discussed in greater detail in a later section.

Community-acquired pneumonia, a leading cause of death globally, occurs in persons with little to no contact with medical settings, such as hospitals or nursing homes, at the time of acquisition. Patients will present with fatigue, dyspnea, cough, fever, chills, and pleuritic chest pain. Diagnosis will be made based upon clinical presentation and chest x-ray films. Antibiotics are the treatment of choice, based on the causative organism. It is important to note that it is often difficult to pin down the exact cause of the pneumonia due to the limited diagnostic methods available at this current time. Antibiotic treatment, as a result, will be based on the clinician's best judgment and empirical evidence.

Hospital-acquired and health care–associated pneumonias occur in patients in medical settings. These patients are likely to have been infected with gram-negative bacilli, such as *Pseudomonas aeruginosa,* and antibiotic-resistant strains, such as *methicillin-resistant Staphylococcus aureus.* Like the other pneumonias, diagnosis is based on clinical presentation and chest x-ray. Treatment is usually a regimen of broad-spectrum antibiotics.

Patients that are immunocompromised, such as those with HIV infection or those undergoing chemotherapy, may be particularly susceptible to pneumonia. Diagnosis is made after blood cultures have been obtained as well as sputum cultures, chest x-ray, and clinical evaluation. Treatment is the same, with special consideration given to the compromised immune function of the patient.

Air-Leak Syndromes

An abnormal leak of air outside of the lung tissue compartments falls into the category of air-leak syndromes. Emphysema, pneumothorax, and subcutaneous emphysema are all examples of air-leak syndromes. Air-leak syndromes are more common in neonates and children.

Air-leak syndromes occur when one or a group of alveoli ruptures and air leaks into the interstitial tissue surrounding the lungs and airways. Other tissues affected include the pleura, mediastinum, subcutaneous tissues, and/or abdominal cavity. This rupture can arise because of blunt force trauma, overdistended lungs, uneven ventilation, or chemical injury, or it may occur idiopathically, spontaneously without a known cause.

Treatment for air-leak syndromes may not be necessary, depending on their severity, as some resolve spontaneously without medical intervention. In some cases, however, the free air that has leaked must be evacuated via chest tube placement. X-ray images will not only diagnose the air leak, but also confirm that it has resolved.

Aspiration

Aspiration pneumonia occurs when a patient inhales something toxic, usually contents of the stomach or something they are eating. Airway obstruction and pneumonia follow aspiration.

Patients with aspiration pneumonia usually have risk factors that the critical care nurse should be aware of before the event occurs, including impaired cognition, impaired swallowing, or GI devices such as a nasogastric tube in place.

A patient who has aspirated may not always exhibit symptoms of aspiration. This is called "silent aspiration" and can go on for some time without any evidence it is occurring. A patient who is silently aspirating may be constantly clearing their throat or have a cough that sounds wet. Symptoms of aspiration, if evident, include fever, discomfort of the chest, coughing while eating and attempting to swallow, and trouble breathing, especially after eating and drinking.

When gastric contents are aspirated, the acidic nature of the stomach acid burns the lining of the airways and lungs. This chemical burn causes immediate bronchoconstriction, swelling, and hemorrhage of the alveoli. This alveolar bursting is what then leads to the associated aspiration pneumonitis.

A patient is diagnosed with aspiration pneumonia after their clinical presentation is evaluated and a chest x-ray is obtained. If silent aspiration is suspected, a barium swallow study may be performed to confirm. Treatment includes antibiotics and removal of the foreign object if possible.

Preventative interventions for aspiration include elevating the head of the patient's bed to at least 30 degrees (90 degrees if the patient is eating). Diet changes may be necessary, including allowing foods that are easy to chew and swallow, discontinuing straw usage for drinks, and monitoring patient eating times. Patients who are at risk for aspiration should not take in fluids through a straw, since the straw shoots fluid directly onto the back of their throat, not allowing a weakened swallow reflex enough time to "catch" it and direct it down the esophagus. The critical care nurse can encourage the patient to tuck their chin while swallowing to ensure food passes into the esophagus rather than the airway.

Chronic Conditions of the Pulmonary System

Many patients that the critical care nurse will encounter will suffer from long-term diseases of the lungs, falling under the category of chronic obstructive pulmonary disease (COPD), asthma, bronchitis, and emphysema. All four chronic conditions overlap in clinical presentation, diagnosis, exacerbations, and treatment, but it is important to know the distinctions between them as well.

COPD is an umbrella term encompassing various chronic lung conditions—such as emphysema, bronchiectasis, chronic bronchitis, certain cases of asthma, or a combination of these—wherein normal breathing is compromised. Thus, it is possible to be diagnosed with COPD but not emphysema, since there are other diseases—namely, chronic bronchitis—that can be at the root of a patient's COPD. A patient diagnosed with COPD often has emphysema and chronic bronchitis together, but this is not necessarily the case. In most cases, COPD is progressive and permanent. Symptoms of COPD include shortness of breath and/or wheezing, chest pain, coughing, and excessive mucus in the airways. Smoking cessation should be encouraged to decrease exacerbations and slow the progression of the disease. Smoking is almost always the cause of emphysema, and therefore, also often heavily involved in causing COPD. Over the course of several years, the disease will worsen, starting with a productive cough and leading to trouble with breathing. Patients with COPD will often complain of a headache that they get every morning. Their chest may become barrel-like in appearance due to hyperinflation of the lungs. Weight loss and muscle wasting are common signs of advanced disease. The patient may breathe with their lips pursed, a sign of "auto-PEEPing." This means they are creating their own PEEP by making the hole their air passes through smaller, like breathing through a straw. As the disease progresses, their exacerbations will increase. An exacerbation is when, for whatever reason—often unknown—their symptoms worsen, and hospitalization often occurs.

Diagnosis of COPD is made based on clinical presentation, pack-a-day history, chest x-ray, and pulmonary function testing. Treatment includes encouragement of smoking cessation, inhaled bronchodilators, corticosteroid use, and supportive care including oxygen therapy and pulmonary rehabilitation.

Asthma is an airway disease in which bronchoconstriction occurs in the airways, usually after some triggering stimuli has set in motion the inflammatory responses of the lung tissue. Patients with asthma will have exacerbations that cause them to have trouble breathing, wheezing, a cough, and tightness in the chest. **Pulsus paradoxus**, or a greater than 10-point fall in systolic BP while breathing in, is a sign of an asthmatic attack, along with tachycardia, tachypnea, and use of accessory muscles to breath.

A diagnosis of asthma will be made based on the patient's clinical presentation, their history of symptoms, and pulmonary function tests. They will be treated with inhaled beta2-agonists and inhaled corticosteroids, as well as monitoring and controlling their exposure to their asthmatic triggers or the substances in their environment that cause exacerbations.

While chronic bronchitis is a hallmark of COPD, acute bronchitis can occur in any patient, most often following an upper respiratory infection (URI). The patient's bronchial tissue has become inflamed because of the URI. The symptoms exhibited are cough, possible fever, and sputum production. A diagnosis of acute bronchitis will be based on clinical presentation, and antibiotics may or may not be used based on the clinician's judgment.

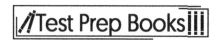

Emphysema usually occurs because of smoking and is defined as a destruction of lung tissue that causes a loss of elasticity, recoil, and alveoli. The airway is more susceptible to collapsing, it hyperinflates, and airflow is limited. Blebs and bullae develop, air trapping occurs, and the airspaces, as a whole, enlarge. All of these physiological effects of emphysema worsen the lungs' functioning capability and can lead to a COPD diagnosis and the exacerbation of such COPD symptoms.

The structural effect of emphysema on alveoli

Normal alveoli

Alveoli

Alveoli with emphysema

Damaged alveoli

Failure to Wean from Mechanical Ventilation

Mechanical ventilation is a means to an end, that end being weaning from ventilation and restoring the patient's full ventilatory capacity and functioning. Weaning from the vent can be a difficult task in some patients, especially if their pulmonary system has been weakened by illness. While the critical care nurse will not oversee vent weaning in most facilities, they are there to support the respiratory care team and physicians in achieving this goal.

Vent weaning is achieved through gradual changes in the level of the patient's dependence on the machine. The respiratory therapy team will likely be performing spontaneous breathing trials on the patient daily, as these have been shown to assist with weaning. This means they turn off the vent and see how the patient does without it for a few breaths. If the patient is completely apneic and oxygen levels immediately drop off, it is not time, and the vent breathing is resumed.

The critical care nurse is aware that sedative and opioid use on the patient over time, though necessary to keep the patient comfortable while on the vent, may end up prolonging the duration of mechanical ventilation. Caution must then be used when sedating the patient, using enough to keep the patient comfortable, but not so much that the patient is "snowed," meaning overly sedated and unable to wean. Halving the dose may be ordered by the doctor, as well as titrating the dose down regularly and performing sedation vacations. **Sedation vacations** mean the nurse turns off sedation for a period of time, usually once a day for an hour or so. Sedation vacation duration also depends on patient tolerance of the procedure.

Pulmonary Fibrosis

Pulmonary fibrosis is a condition in which lung tissue begins to scar, becoming thick and stiff. This noncompliant tissue leads to issues with the patient's ability to breathe. Most cases of pulmonary fibrosis are idiopathic, meaning they have no known cause.

Idiopathic pulmonary fibrosis (IPF) may arise because of genetic factors, but environmental or factors yet to be discovered may also play into its development. For whatever reason, the cells of the alveoli stop functioning in an appropriate manner and turn into scar tissue rather than healthy tissue. These cells then begin to exhibit a honeycomb pattern when examined via microscope.

A patient with IPF will likely present with cough, complaints of dyspnea on exertion, and fine crackles that sound like Velcro being pulled apart on auscultation of the bases. The patient's lungs, on suspicion of IPF, will likely be imaged using CT scanning. A biopsy may be taken of lung tissue to visualize the cells and look for scar tissue.

The patient diagnosed with IPF has a poor prognosis, with 3 years or less to live after diagnosis. Treatment may include antifibrotics, oxygen therapy, and supportive care.

Pulmonary Hypertension

When the pressure in the pulmonary circulation rises, it is termed **pulmonary hypertension**. The blood vessels within the pulmonary beds of circulation become constricted and sometimes even obstructed. This raised BP may cause failure of the right ventricle of the heart.

Causes of pulmonary hypertension may be idiopathic, but left heart failure, diastolic dysfunction, parenchymal lung disease, and a PE have been known to raise the pulmonary pressures.

A patient with pulmonary hypertension may complain of exertional dyspnea and chronic fatigue, experience loss of consciousness, and feel chest discomfort. Diagnosis is made via echocardiography, which estimates the pressures, and confirmed by right heart catheterization.

Pulmonary hypertension can be treated through use of vasodilators and diuretics. Sildenafil is an example of a phosphodiesterase inhibitor used to treat pulmonary hypertension and is helpful in increasing blood flow in the lungs. Amlodipine is an example of a calcium channel blocker, a class of drugs that may be helpful for pulmonary hypertension. Epoprostenol is a drug specifically formulated for use in patients with pulmonary hypertension. Lung transplantation may be an option in advanced disease states.

Status Asthmaticus

Acute severe asthma attacks, also known as **status asthmaticus**, are repeated, back-to-back asthma attacks that are not responding to the usual treatment of bronchodilators. Status asthmaticus is an emergency that requires special medical treatment to resolve.

A patient experiencing a severe asthma attack that is unresponsive to bronchodilators may have chest tightness, severe shortness of breath, a dry cough, and wheezing. Their airway is undergoing bronchospasm, inflammation, and mucus plugging, all of which contribute to difficulty breathing. The patient's lungs may be retaining carbon dioxide, resulting in hypoxemia and respiratory failure.

Often a respiratory illness is the triggering factor in status asthmaticus, occurring a few days before the attack. This weakens the body's immune defenses, leading to exacerbation of asthma. Other triggers may include exposure to allergens or irritants in the environment with an especially potent effect.

In the emergency treatment of a patient with status asthmaticus, subcutaneous epinephrine may be used. Alternatively, terbutaline may be used, as it has fewer cardiac effects such as tachycardia. Albuterol that has been nebulized may be administered alongside nebulized ipratropium. Corticosteroids such as prednisone should be given to decrease the systemic inflammatory response. If a bacterial infection seems to be part of the patient's presentation, antibiotics may be used. Supplemental oxygen will be part of the patient's therapy as well.

If the patient is unresponsive to all the above treatments and respiratory function continues to decline, noninvasive positive pressure ventilation or mechanical ventilation will be considered to stabilize the patient, restore ventilation and oxygenation, and prevent further complications such as cardiac arrest.

Thoracic Surgery

In certain conditions of the lung, thoracic surgery may be considered. A thoracic surgeon is one who specializes in operations on the thoracic region of the body, involving the organs of the chest. The heart and lungs are the primary targets of these surgical procedures.

Surgeries may be performed to remove cancerous tumors of the lung. Possible procedures a patient would undergo for this purpose would be a pneumonectomy, lobectomy, wedge resection, or sleeve resection. **Pneumonectomy** removes the entire lung. **Lobectomy** removes the entire lobe containing the cancerous tumor. **Wedge resection** removes part of the affected lobe. **Sleeve resection** refers to "trimming" the affected part of the airway and sewing it back together, like cutting a stain off a sleeve and reattaching the upper and lower portions.

If a thoracic surgeon wishes to visualize the interior of the chest wall and surrounding tissues, they may opt to perform a thoracoscopy. During this procedure, small incisions are made into the chest wall, and a thin tube with a camera at the end, called a **scope,** is inserted. The surgeon then explores the interior cavity and visualizes the area they wish to view. This procedure may be used to biopsy tissue for histological analysis. A more invasive procedure used to visualize the interior chest cavity is called a **thoracotomy,** where the chest is opened directly.

Thoracic Trauma

A thoracic trauma can be summarized as an injury to the chest. Frequently, chest trauma results in death within the first few minutes or hours after injury, due to the vitality of the heart and lungs caged within the thoracic cavity. When these organs are damaged, aggressive intervention is necessary to save lives.

A short list of common thoracic traumas includes hemothorax, pneumothorax, disruption of the aorta, flail chest, blunt cardiac injury, pulmonary contusion, and cardiac tamponade. Bone injuries may also occur, such as cracked ribs, clavicle fractures, and fractures of the sternum and scapula.

Hemothorax and pneumothorax may occur at the same time due to their proximity to one another. Hemothorax is a condition in which blood is hemorrhaging and begins filling the pleural space. Pneumothorax occurs when there is an unsealed opening in the thoracic wall, disrupting normal airflow and ventilation. The larger the hole, the worse the respiratory distress and failure. Patients with pneumothorax may have a wound that makes a sucking sound, indicating air moving through an abnormal pathway.

Multiple rib fractures may cause a separating of the chest wall from the thoracic cage, resulting in a disruption to the patient's ability to inspire air. **Flail chest,** the term for this condition, is caused by a blunt force trauma in most cases, which in turn causes significant pulmonary contusion beneath the site of the chest wall separation.

Cardiac tamponade describes the condition in which blood surrounds the pericardial sac, decreasing the heart's ability to fill. Patients experience hypotension, jugular vein distention, and muffled heart tones upon auscultation. A pericardiocentesis is immediately necessary, in which a needle is inserted and the leaked blood aspirated, to relieve pressure surrounding the heart and normalize BP.

Blunt chest injuries may cause a rib fracture. Rib fractures often occur simultaneously with other thoracic trauma, such as pneumothorax, flail chest, hemothorax, and tracheobronchial injuries. A rib fracture on its own is painful, but it is not complicated, nor does it need much treatment besides analgesia. Analgesia is achieved using opioids and possibly concurrent NSAID use.

Tracheal perforation refers to a tear in the upper airway of the pulmonary tree. Thoracic trauma may be the cause of a tracheal perforation, but it may also have occurred during a medical procedure such as endotracheal intubation or bronchoscopy. Surgical repair will be necessary to repair the tear after it has been confirmed using CT scanning and chest x-ray.

Practice Questions

19/26 = 73.07%

1. Which category of pulmonary emboli entails impairment of right ventricular function as well as severe hypotension?
    a. Small ∅
    b. Submassive *RV function impaired w/out hypotension*
    c. Massive *RV function impaired / hypotension*
    d. Grand *∅ category*

2. When attempting to diagnose a PE in a patient with renal failure, which type of scan will likely be performed?
    a. Transesophageal echocardiography *∅ back of heart*
    b. CT scan with contrast *∅ w/ renal failure*
    c. MRI of the thoracic cage *∅ appropriate*
    d. V/Q scan *ventilation/perfusion of lungs visualized*

3. Which of the following is NOT a way in which mechanical ventilation benefits the patient?
    a. Creates alkalotic state of the blood. *∅ alk/acid are beneficial*
    b. Decreases the work of breathing.
    c. Increases cardiac output.
    d. Creates positive end-expiratory pressure (PEEP).
    (+)

4. Which of the following is not a usual drug of choice when providing analgesia to the mechanically ventilated patient?
    a. Morphine
    b. Dopamine *maintain BP*
    c. Fentanyl
    d. Propofol

5. Patients on the cusp of respiratory failure may exhibit which of the following early signs and symptoms?
    a. Decreased respiratory rate
    b. Unconsciousness   *late signs*
    c. Cyanosis
    d. Agitation *w/ confusion, oxygen hunger*

6. Which of the following is not an example of a drug that may cause respiratory failure in higher doses or in sensitive patients?
    a. Morphine
    b. Hydrocodone
    c. Naloxone *antidote*
    d. Alprazolam

7. What is the most common bacterial cause of pneumonias in patients?
    a. *Streptococcus pneumoniae* ✱ *most common*
    b. *Klebsiella pneumoniae*
    c. *Chlamydophila pneumoniae*
    d. *Mycoplasma pneumoniae*

49

8. Which category of pneumonia is more likely to occur in a patient who is undergoing chemotherapy for a metastatic lung cancer?

    a. Community acquired — *ø contact w/ medical facilities*

    b. Hospital acquired *hospitalized / ↓ mobility*

    c. Immunocompromised *weakened immune, HIV/chemo*

    d. Health care associated *long term hospl facilities*

9. Which of the following is not an example of an air-leak syndrome?

    a. Emphysema

    b. Pneumothorax

    c. Subcutaneous emphysema

    d. Flail chest *rib fx, separation of chest wall from rib cage*

10. Which of the following is not a common cause of air-leak syndromes?

    a. Obstruction of blood vessels *causes ischemia, ø rupture*

    b. Blunt force trauma

    c. Chemical injury

    d. Overdistention of lungs

11. A patient who is silently aspirating may exhibit which of the following signs and symptoms?

    a. Flat, red rash on the thoracic region ø

    b. Constant clearing of the throat

    c. Swollen lymph nodes on the neck *URI*

    d. Trouble remembering person, place, and time *precurssor*

12. What intervention should the nurse do to prevent aspiration?

    a. Encourage early mobilization after the surgical procedure.

    b. Allow straw use in drinks to increase the patient's fluid intake.

    c. Instruct the patient to tilt their head back when swallowing.

    d. Elevate the head of the bed to 90 degrees while the patient is eating.

13. Which of the following is a common symptom of COPD?

    a. Dry cough *cough normally productive*

    b. Morning headache

    c. Narrow chest

    d. Weight gain

14. Which of the following actions by a patient with COPD creates their own positive end-expiratory pressure?

    a. Tri-pod posing

    b. Wide open-mouth breathing

    c. Pursed-lip breathing *straw-like breathing creates PEEP*

    d. Frequent coughing

15. Which of the following is not a result of emphysema?

    a. Blebs — *characterized by blebs, bullae*

    b. Air trapping *air trapping, air space enlarge*

    c. Air space enlargement

    d. Bronchoconstriction *= asthma*

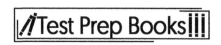

16. Daily breaks from sedation in the mechanically ventilated patient are commonly called what?
    a. Sedation vacation
    b. Spontaneous breathing trial
    c. Vent weaning
    d. Analgesia arrest

17. Apnea and loss of normal oxygenation during a spontaneous breathing trial are signs that what should occur?
    a. Sedation should be increased.
    b. The breathing trial should continue for a few more minutes.
    c. An antidote for respiratory distress should be administered.
    d. Mechanical ventilation should continue. *Ø ready to breathe on own*

18. Pulmonary fibrosis leads to all but which of the following conditions of the lung tissue?
    a. Increased stiffness
    b. Increased scar tissue
    c. Increased compliance = *↓ compliance, Ø inc*
    d. Increased thickness

19. Which of the following is not characteristic of a patient with pulmonary fibrosis and their clinical presentation?
    a. Auscultation of wheezing in the upper airways *asthma*
    b. Dyspnea upon exertion
    c. Auscultation of Velcro-like sounds in the bases of the lungs
    d. "Honeycomb" appearance of tissue upon histological analysis

20. Which of the following procedures confirms a diagnosis of pulmonary hypertension?
    a. Transesophageal echocardiography
    b. Right cardiac catheterization *(swan, RHC, confirms)*
    c. Left cardiac catherization
    d. Lung transplantation

21. Pulmonary hypertension will likely be treated with all but which of the following drug therapies?
    a. Sildenafil
    b. Amlodipine
    c. Epoprostenol
    d. Diazepam

22. Which of the following terms refers to severe bronchoconstriction with wheezing that does not respond to the usual bronchodilation treatment?
    a. *Delirium tremens*
    b. *Status asthmaticus*
    c. *Pulsus paradoxus*
    d. *Febre rubra*

23. Which of the following medications administered during status asthmaticus targets the systemic inflammation being experienced by the patient?
    a. Inhaled bronchodilators
    b. Subcutaneous epinephrine   *direct*
    c. Nebulized albuterol
    d. Oral corticosteroids   *systemic*

24. Which of the following surgeries performed by a cardiothoracic surgeon removes a section of an airway leading to the lung, sewing together the top and bottom of the section removed?
    a. Pneumonectomy
    b. Lobectomy
    c. Sleeve resection   *affected airway removed*
    d. Wedge resection   *and top/bottom sewn together*

25. Which of the following is a more invasive procedure performed by a thoracic surgeon involving opening the chest wall to visualize the interior structures?
    a. Thoracotomy
    b. Thoracocentesis
    c. Thoracobronchotomy
    d. Thoracoscopy

26. What emergency surgery is necessary to relieve cardiac tamponade?
    a. Thoracocentesis
    b. Pericardiocentesis
    c. Left heart cardiac catheterization
    d. Open heart surgery

Answer Explanations

1. C: A massive pulmonary embolism impairs right ventricular function as well as causing marked hypotension. Small does not affect the right ventricular function or blood pressure. Submassive affects the right ventricle without hypotension. Grand is not a category of a PE.

2. D: A patient with a suspected PE that is in renal failure will likely undergo V/Q scanning, in which ventilation and perfusion of the lungs are visualized. Transesophageal echocardiography is used for visualizing the back of the heart and is not appropriate in this scenario. CT scanning with contrast is contraindicated, as the patient with renal failure cannot tolerate the dye, which is primarily metabolized by the kidney. MRI is not an appropriate scan for a PE, or at least not a usual scan.

3. A: Mechanical ventilation is likely to create an acidotic state in the blood, rather than alkalotic. Neither acidotic or alkalotic states are particularly beneficial for the patient but may be tolerated for a time with the greater good of oxygenation and perfusion being maintained until the patient is stable. Mechanical ventilation decreases the work of breathing, increases cardiac output, and creates positive end-expiratory pressure (PEEP) for a patient so they might rest until they are stabilized and can be weaned from the vent.

4. B: Dopamine is a commonly infused drug in a mechanically ventilated patient, but not for the purpose of analgesia. Rather, it is used to maintain a normal blood pressure in a hemodynamically unstable patient. The usual drugs of choice include morphine, fentanyl, and propofol. These three are commonly used to provide analgesia to a mechanically ventilated patient.

5. D: An early sign of respiratory distress is agitation, along with confusion and oxygen hunger. Later signs of respiratory distress occur when the patient has become fatigued because of the respiratory effort they have put forth. These signs include decreased respiratory rate, unconsciousness, and cyanosis.

6. C: Naloxone, or Narcan, is the antidote for respiratory depression caused by an opioid overdose. Morphine and hydrocodone are examples of opioids that might cause respiratory failure if overdose occurs. Alprazolam is an example of a benzodiazepine, a known cause of respiratory failure if overdosed.

7. A: *Streptococcus pneumoniae* is the most common cause of bacterial pneumonia. The other three organisms listed are also bacteria and may cause pneumonia if they infect the lungs, but not as commonly as *S. pneumoniae.*

8. C: Immunocompromised pneumonia occurs in patients whose immune systems have been weakened. It may occur in patients who have an HIV infection or are undergoing chemotherapy or radiation regimens. Community-acquired pneumonia occurs in persons who had little to no contact with medical facilities prior to the infection. Hospital-acquired pneumonias occur in patients who have been hospitalized and as a result of immobilization. Health care-associated pneumonias occur in patients in long-term facilities or some other health care facility besides a hospital.

9. D: Flail chest is not an example of an air-leak syndrome. Flail chest occurs because of rib fracture, which then causes separation of the chest wall from the rib cage. This is a medical emergency and may be associated with pneumothorax, an example of an air-leak syndrome. Emphysema and subcutaneous emphysema are both examples of air-leak syndromes.

10. A: Obstruction of blood vessels causes ischemia in tissues, not alveolar rupture, which leads to air-leak syndromes. Common causes of air-leak syndromes include blunt force trauma, chemical injury, overdistention of lungs, or uneven ventilation. They can also arise spontaneously, called idiopathic.

11. B: Constant clearing of the throat is a sign that a patient is silently aspirating. Integument symptoms such as rash are not associated with this condition. Swollen lymph nodes on the neck indicate possible upper respiratory infection. Neurological deficits such as memory and orientation loss are not associated with silent aspiration, but may occur because of stroke, which is a precursor to difficulty swallowing in some cases.

12. D: Elevating the head of the bed to 90 degrees is the best option on this list, as it helps keep the patient upright while they eat, which aids swallowing. Early mobilization is good for all patients, but for the purpose of preventing blood clots and deconditioning, not specifically for helping prevent aspiration. Drinking straws are an aspiration risk, as they shoot fluid directly onto the back of the patient's throat, not allowing a patient with dysphagia enough time to properly swallow. The chin-tuck maneuver—not tilting the head backward—is the recommended tip to give to patients to assist with swallowing.

13. B: A morning headache is a common symptom of COPD. The cough associated with COPD is usually productive. A barrel chest, not a narrowed chest, is common due to hyperinflation of the lungs. Patients with COPD will often experience weight loss and muscle wasting because of the disease.

14. C: Pursed-lip breathing, breathing through a small, straw-like opening of the mouth, creates positive end-expiratory pressure (PEEP) for the patient with compromised lung function, as is the case with COPD patients. Tri-pod breathing is common in COPD patients but does not increase PEEP; rather, it creates more space for lung volume when they are having trouble breathing. Wide open-mouth breathing is not helpful for increasing PEEP. Frequent coughing is caused by the body's constant mucociliary response to try and clear mucus from inflamed airways.

15. D: Emphysema is a destruction of lung tissue that is characterized by the development of blebs and bullae, air trapping, and overall air space enlargement. Bronchoconstriction is a cause of asthmatic attacks and is not specifically associated with emphysema.

16. A: *Sedation vacation* is the term used to describe giving the patient a break from analgesia with the purpose of preventing over-sedation and encouraging eventual vent weaning. Spontaneous breathing trial may occur during the sedation vacation but does not refer to the practice specifically. Analgesia arrest implies a break from sedation but is not a commonly used term.

17. D: If a patient becomes apneic and oxygenation drops off during a spontaneous breathing trial, it is a sign that the patient should be placed back on mechanical ventilation, as they are not ready to breathe on their own. Increasing the sedation will worsen the patient's breathing function. Continuing the breathing trial will lead to organ damage due to lack of oxygenation and perfusion. An antidote is not appropriate in this scenario.

18. C: Increased compliance of lung tissue is not a sign of pulmonary fibrosis. Pulmonary fibrosis is characterized by increased stiffness, scarring, and thickness of lung tissue, often arising from idiopathic causes, and instead decreases lung compliance.

19. A: Wheezing that is heard in the upper airways is characteristic of asthma, not pulmonary fibrosis. The scarring of the lung tissue that occurs in pulmonary fibrosis causes the patient to become dyspneic upon exertion. The nurse will often hear fine crackles in the bases of the lungs that sound like Velcro being pulled apart. Upon histological analysis of the lung tissue, the cells will appear to form a honeycomblike configuration.

20. B: Right cardiac catheterization is a procedure that will confirm a diagnosis of pulmonary hypertension. Transesophageal echocardiography is useful in visualizing the back side of the heart but does not fit with this specific scenario. Left cardiac catheterization enters the opposite side of the heart and is not helpful in confirming diagnosis. Lung transplantation is a surgical procedure used to treat severe cases of pulmonary hypertension.

21. D: Diazepam is an anxiolytic that is not specifically used for the treatment of pulmonary hypertension. Diuretics, calcium channel blockers, and vasodilators may all be used to treat pulmonary hypertension. Sildenafil is an example of a phosphodiesterase inhibitor and is helpful in increasing blood flow in the lungs. Amlodipine is an example of a calcium channel blocker, a class of drugs that can be helpful for pulmonary hypertension. Epoprostenol is a drug specifically formulated for use in patients with pulmonary hypertension.

22. B: *Status asthmaticus* is the Latin term for a severe asthma attack, characterized by wheezing and bronchoconstriction, that is unresponsive to the usual therapy of bronchodilators. *Delirium tremens* is the set of symptoms experienced by an alcoholic in withdrawal. *Pulsus paradoxus* is defined as a drop in the systolic blood pressure by ten points and a decrease in the amplitude of pulse waves while the patient breathes in. It can be observed during cardiac tamponade. *Febre rubra* is the Latin term for scarlet fever.

23. D: The big hint here is the route of administration: Oral corticosteroids will pass through the gastrointestinal tract, where they will be absorbed into the systemic circulation in the small intestine, affecting the body system as a whole. Inhaled and nebulized drugs such as bronchodilators and albuterol will directly affect the inflamed airways of status asthmaticus, thus not affecting systemic inflammation. The same goes for epinephrine administered subcutaneously. Its action will primarily be targeting the airways, with bronchodilation being the desired effect.

24. C: Sleeve resection is the correct answer, referring to a thoracic surgery in which an affected part of the airway is removed with the top and bottom sections being sewn together. This action is similar to cutting a stain off a sleeve and reattaching the top and bottom sections of the sleeve back together—hence, the name "sleeve resection." Pneumonectomy is the removal of an entire lung. Lobectomy is the removal of a lobe. Wedge resection refers to removing a part of an affected lobe.

25. A: A thoracotomy is the opening of the chest by a thoracic surgeon to visualize the interior structures and tissue of the chest. Thoracocentesis is an invasive procedure where small incisions are made in the chest wall with the purpose of removing air or fluid and inserting a chest tube to drain. Thoracocentesis is also called a pleural tap. Thoracobronchotomy is a procedure where an incision is made into the bronchus and thorax, usually to remove a tumor or foreign object. Thoracoscopy is a less invasive procedure involving small incisions and the insertion of a thin tube with a camera affixed to the end, called a scope, to visualize the interior structure and tissues of the chest.

26. B: Pericardiocentesis is indicated in the emergent situation of cardiac tamponade. A needle is inserted, and the hemorrhaging blood is aspirated from the pericardial sac. Thoracocentesis, or pleural tap, can be used for hemothorax or pneumothorax. Left cardiac catherization is used in acute myocardial infarctions to open obstructed coronary vessels. Open heart surgery can be performed in emergency situations involving thoracic trauma, but not specifically for cardiac tamponade.

Endocrine/Hematology/Gastrointestinal/Renal/Integumentary

The critical care nurse will encounter several conditions affecting the hormonal regulation of the human body, the blood and its unique chemistry, the digestive tract, the kidneys and their filtrative processes, and the largest organ of the body, the skin, which protects the interior of the body from the exterior environment. This section comprises a discussion of those body systems, including the endocrine, hematological, gastrointestinal, renal, and integumentary systems.

Endocrine

The hormones of the body play a key role in metabolism and the regulation of body processes. Each hormone, produced in various glands throughout the body, has a specific target tissue that it acts upon, producing a specific result. Dysfunction of hormonal regulation can lead to disease states, as will be discussed in the section on the next page.

Major Human Endocrine Glands and Some of Their Hormones

Gland		Hormone	Chemical Class	Representative Actions	Regulated By
Hypothalamus		Hormones released from the posterior pituitary and hormones that regulate the anterior pituitary *see below*			
Posterior pituitary gland *Releases neurohormones made in hypothalamus*		Oxytocin	Peptide	Stimulates contraction of uterus and mammary gland cells	Nervous system
		Antidiuretic hormone **ADH**	Peptide	Promotes retention of water by kidneys	Water/salt balance
Anterior pituitary gland		Growth hormone **GH**	Protein	Stimulates growth (especially bones) and metabolic functions	Hypothalamic hormones
		Prolactin **PRL**	Protein	Stimulates milk production and secretion	Hypothalamic hormones
		Follicle-stimulating hormone **FSH**	Glycoprotein	Stimulates production of ova and sperm	Hypothalamic hormones
		Luteinizing hormone **LH**	Glycoprotein	Stimulates ovaries and testes	Hypothalamic hormones
		Thyroid-stimulating hormone **TSH**	Glycoprotein	Stimulates thyroid gland	Hypothalamic hormones
		Adrenocorticotropic hormone **ACTH**	Peptide	Stimulates adrenal cortex to secrete glucocorticoids	Hypothalamic hormones
Thyroid gland		Triiodothyrocine T_3 Thyrocine T_2	Amine	Stimulate and maintain metabolic processes	TSH
		Calcitonine	Peptide	Lowers blood calcium level	Calcium in blood
Parathyroid glands		Parathyroid hormone **PTH**	Peptide	Raises blood calcium level	Calcium in blood
Pancreas		Insulin	Protein	Lowers blood glucose level	Glucose in blood
		Glucagon	Protein	Raises blood insulin level	Glucose in blood
Adrenal glands	*Adrenal medulla*	Epinephrine Norepinephrine	Amines	Raises blood glucose level; Increases metabolic activities; Constrict certain blood vessels	Nervous system
	Adrenal cortex	Glucocorticoids	Steroid	Raises blood glucose level	ACTH
		Mineralocorticoids	Steroid	Promote reabsorbtion of Na^+ and excretion of K^+ in kidneys	K^+ in blood; angiotensin II
Gonads	*Testes*	Androgens	Steroid	Support sperm formation; Promote development and maintenance of male secondary sex characteristics	FSH LH
	Ovaries	Estrogens	Steroid	Stimulate uterine lining growth; Promote development and maintenance of female secondary sex characteristics	FSH LH
		Progestins	Steroid	Promote uterine lining growth;	FSH and LH
Pineal gland		Melatonin	Amine	Involved in biological rhythms	Light/dark cycles

Acute Hypoglycemia

In the body, a normal amount of blood glucose is necessary as an energy source for metabolic processes. The brain relies on glucose as an energy source to perform its functions. The term "blood sugar" refers to the amount of glucose circulating in one's blood at any given time. A normal blood sugar before a person eats falls into the 70 mg/dl to 99 mg/dl range. After one eats, blood sugar rises, but should be no more than 140 mg/dl a few hours after a meal. When the blood glucose level falls below 50 mg/dl, this is considered hypoglycemia, or low blood sugar.

Hypoglycemia may occur with or without symptoms. The body has a number of regulatory activities that are performed to correct low blood sugar. As a compensatory mechanism, the levels of glucagon and epinephrine may rise, and growth hormone and cortisol levels may increase. These regulatory mechanisms may occur and correct the hypoglycemia before any noticeable symptoms arise.

Symptoms of hypoglycemia are reflective of the autonomic activity occurring within the body. The patient may be sweating, feel warm, or experience nausea, anxiety, and palpitations. The patient may be trembling, complain of headache, experience blurry or double vision, become confused, slur their speech, or even begin to have a seizure or enter a comatose state. Many of these symptoms are caused by the lack of blood glucose to the brain, causing neurological symptoms.

The cause of an acute hypoglycemic state is almost always drug-induced, especially if the patient is receiving insulin therapy. Overtreatment with insulin without proper balance with the patient's mealtime schedule will result in hypoglycemia. Patients in the hospital setting often fall victim to hypoglycemia due to an ever-changing schedule of tests, procedures, and periods of time where they are required to fast.

Treatment of hypoglycemia usually includes administration of dextrose or some other form of sugar. Oral glucagon is an option in the alert patient who can swallow. Symptoms should be corrected upon normalization of blood sugar.

Diabetes Insipidus

Vasopressin, also known as the antidiuretic hormone, is made in the hypothalamus within the brain and stored in the pituitary gland. It is then secreted by the pituitary gland, targeting the tissue of the kidneys and blood vessels. The role of vasopressin is to help the body concentrate urine and maintain a healthy balance of fluid within the blood.

When the pituitary does not produce enough vasopressin, the kidneys' ability to concentrate urine is significantly decreased, to the point of massive fluid loss through urination.

The term "antidiuretic hormone" should give one a clue as to how this disease works; if the hormone that is supposed to prevent diuresis is inhibited, then severe diuresis will occur.

The condition that results from the inhibition of vasopressin is called "diabetes insipidus." The onset of the disease may happen slowly over time or quite abruptly. The patient will usually present with symptoms of enormous fluid intake and copious quantities of urine production, termed **polydipsia** and **polyuria**, respectively.

The urine produced by individuals with diabetes insipidus is quite diluted, due to a lack of concentration ability of the kidneys. The patient will require volume replenishment as soon as possible, to prevent further complications of dehydration and hypovolemia.

Since it is difficult clinically to perform tests to detect the amount of vasopressin within the body, the test most often used for diabetes insipidus is the water-deprivation test. The patient is carefully monitored while fasting from fluids. Urine output is monitored and analyzed for osmolality and electrolyte concentrations. Toward the end of the testing, vasopressin is administered and the effect it has on the urine measured. If the patient is responsive to the vasopressin and there are signs that without it the urine becomes overly diluted, it is probable that the patient has diabetes insipidus.

Differential diagnoses to be mindful of in a patient with diabetes insipidus are diabetes mellitus and psychogenic polydipsia. A patient with diabetes mellitus, a condition in which insulin regulation of blood glucose is impaired, may present with polyuria like the polyuria present in diabetes insipidus. Patients with psychogenic polydipsia take in enormous quantities of water but not for the same reason as a patient with diabetes insipidus. Their water intake is due to an emotional disturbance or mental illness such as schizophrenia. The critical care nurse will be mindful of this when assessing patients with symptoms of polydipsia and polyuria.

Diabetic Ketoacidosis

A patient diagnosed with diabetes mellitus may be prone to a complication of this condition called diabetic ketoacidosis (DKA). The process of developing DKA is a complex metabolic pathway in which the body seeks alternative energy sources to glucose and an acidotic state results.

At the beginning of DKA, the body is in a state of insulin deficiency. This can happen as a result of diabetes mellitus, and the body must compensate to continue operations as usual. The body begins to metabolize triglycerides and amino acids to create energy. In a normal state, the body breaks down glucose as an energy source. However, when insulin is deficient and blood glucose supply is in flux all the time, as is the case with diabetes mellitus, the body searches for alternatives.

The breakdown of triglycerides and amino acids then causes an increase in serum levels of glycerol and free fatty acids as a byproduct of lipolysis, or fat breakdown. Alanine also rises in the serum as a byproduct of muscle breakdown, as another energy source when the body cannot find enough glucose. This rise in alanine and glycerol stimulate the liver to produce its own glucose as an energy source. Glucagon, which is produced in the pancreas and used as an emergency source of energy when outside glucose sources drop, rises to excessive levels and stimulates free fatty acids to be converted to ketones. This process is called **ketogenesis** and is normally blocked by sufficient levels of insulin. Ketogenesis results in ketoacids, such as acetone, which create the acidic environment of DKA. Acetone is released from the body by way of respiration, which is why a patient with DKA has a "fruity" smell to their breath.

When the blood sugar rises during DKA, this causes substantial amounts of fluids to be excreted through the urine, called **osmotic diuresis**. This leads to fluid and electrolyte imbalances. Potassium levels must be carefully monitored during DKA. They may not initially fall in serum tests because, despite great loss of potassium through the urine, there is also a great release of potassium from the cells into the blood stream. Potassium will be ushered back into the cells when insulin levels return to normal.

Presenting symptoms of DKA include polyuria, polydipsia, nausea, and abdominal pain. Diagnosis will be made based on symptoms and measurements of arterial blood gases. Presence of ketones in the blood stream, an anion gap of >12, and a pH of < 7.30 are considered positive diagnostic signs of DKA.

Treatment of DKA will include insulin administration, correction of fluid and electrolyte imbalances, and possibly bicarbonate to correct severe cases of acidosis.

Hyperglycemia

Hyperglycemia, or a random blood sugar reading not affected by a recent meal that is greater than 200 mg/dL, is often a symptom of insulin resistance or insulin deficiency. Insulin resistance and deficiency are the key factors producing diabetes types I and II, hence hyperglycemia is a trademark of these two diseases.

When insulin does not properly regulate the level of blood glucose circulating, blood sugar rises to unhealthy levels. This produces a sequela of complications, as well as some unpleasant symptoms in the patient experiencing hyperglycemia.

The most commonly-associated symptoms of hyperglycemia are polydipsia and polyuria, in which a person is drinking and then urinating copious amounts of fluids. A patient might also experience nausea, warmth, and blurred vision. The high level of circulating blood sugar puts the patient at risk for bacterial and fungal infections, as these organisms feed on and thrive in environments where there are high levels of glucose.

Prolonged polyuria will result in dehydration, as evidenced by tachycardia, hypotension, fatigue, and weakness in the patient. These are serious complications that will be treated with fluid resuscitation and electrolyte correction if imbalances exist. High blood glucose will be treated with insulin therapy, including oral antihyperglycemics, and injectable glucagon.

Hyperglycemic Hyperosmolar Nonketotic Syndrome (HHNK)

A patient with Type II diabetes still produces insulin, though insulin response and efficacy is limited as the cells have developed a resistance to insulin. When blood sugar rises to unhealthy levels, it stimulates the kidneys to drop large amounts of urine, a condition called polyuria. The blood volume is thus depleted, causing a state of dehydration and abnormal concentration of the blood. Concentration of the blood creates a hyperosmolar state in the blood stream. When the blood is concentrated yet not acidotic as a result of fat cells breaking down, this is called hyperglycemic hyperosmolar nonketotic syndrome.

HHNK can result from a patient not taking their prescribed diabetic medications appropriately, causing a hyperglycemic state. At other times, an infection or illness unrelated to diabetes mellitus may cause a hyperglycemic state. Corticosteroids are known to cause a rise in blood sugar, thus their use must be administered with caution. If the patient also suffers from high blood sugar and has been prescribed diuretics, this may also cause a hyperosmolar state.

The concentrated blood of HHNK will primarily cause neurological deficits such as confusion, disorientation, drowsiness, and even coma. Certain patients will experience seizures or stroke-like syndromes. Death may occur if HHNK is left untreated.

HHNK will be diagnosed based on symptoms of confusion and blood tests to look for hyperosmolarity of the blood, as well as decreased blood volume signaling dehydration. Treatment will occur via intravenous (IV) therapy to correct fluid and electrolyte imbalances.

Syndrome of Inappropriate Secretion of Antidiuretic Hormone (SIADH)

Antidiuretic hormone, or vasopressin, is released by the pituitary gland to signal the kidneys to retain fluid in the body. When too much vasopressin is released, as is the case in SIADH, fluid is retained and sodium levels become diluted, resulting in hyponatremia.

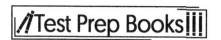

SIADH may occur in some cases of cancer where vasopressin is being produced outside of its normal pituitary gland location. Hospitalized and elderly populations are also susceptible to SIADH.

A patient with SIADH will present with confusion and fatigue, common hyponatremic symptoms. Diagnosis will be made based on clinical presentation and after analysis of blood tests, which will uncover the hyponatremia.

Fluid intake will be restricted to prevent further volume dilution. Hypertonic saline, which has a high concentration of sodium, will be used to correct the hyponatremia. Drugs that reduce the effects of vasopressin may be used, such as demeclocycline or lithium.

Hematology/Immunology

Anemia

There are certain components in the blood that have the capacity to carry oxygen to the tissues of the body. These components are called the red blood cells (RBCs), hematocrit, and hemoglobin. When any of these three components drops in number, oxygen-carrying capacity also drops. A hemoglobin of less than 14 g/dL, a hematocrit of less than 42%, or a red blood cell count of less than 3.4 million/mL are all general ranges of what is considered anemic.

Often anemia is not a disease in and of itself but rather a symptom of an underlying disorder. The practitioner will investigate for underlying causes of anemia to make sure nothing is missed.

There are three broad categories of anemias, not including blood loss: microcytic anemias, normocytic anemias, and macrocytic anemias. In microcytic anemias, including iron-transport deficiency, lead poisoning, and thalassemia, the heme and globin synthesis is defective or deficient. Testing for microcytic anemias will include an analysis of the patient's iron stores. In normocytic anemias, the RBC is normal in size but deficient in number. Examples of normocytic anemias include anemia of chronic disease and aplastic anemia acquired from primary bone marrow disorders. Macrocytic anemias, caused by abnormal DNA synthesis, lead to large RBCs that do not have sufficient oxygen-carrying ability.

The commonly-seen symptoms in a patient with anemia include fatigue, weakness, difficulty breathing during exercise, and a pale skin tone. Pallor, or paleness, can be assessed in a dark-skinned patient by looking at the bottoms of his/her feet, palms, lips, buccal mucosa, and conjunctiva of the eye. Dark-skinned patients will usually have a warm tone, but when anemic or cyanotic, they will have a more gray or ashen hue.

As mentioned, there are a variety of different types of anemias. Thalassemia, common in those of Mediterranean descent, is one type in which the amount of oxygen-carrying hemoglobin is decreased causing pallor, weakness, fatigue, and poor growth. Folate deficiency anemia, associated with alcoholism, is a result of poor absorption of nutrients and decreases the amount of folate available to RBCs, thus decreasing oxygen delivery to tissues. Infections, cancers, and many other illnesses may destroy RBCs, hemoglobin, and/or hematocrit, causing an anemia.

The treatment of anemia will depend on the underlying cause and the patient's symptomology. If the patient is anemic because of massive blood loss, blood transfusions will be required. If the anemia is caused by deficient erythropoiesis, the process by which blood is formed, drugs like erythropoietin will be used to stimulate blood production.

Coagulopathies

Coagulation is the process by which the blood clots to prevent excessive bleeding when an injury occurs. The process of coagulation is orchestrated by several different components of the blood. Injury first occurs, followed by action from the platelets, activation of proteins and a cascade of other coagulation components, conversion of prothrombin to thrombin, then fibrinogen to fibrin, and finally hemostasis, or stopping of bleeding, is achieved.

When a step in this complicated process is interrupted and hemostasis is not adequately achieved and disease arises, it is called a **coagulopathy**. Idiopathic thrombocytopenia purpura (ITP), disseminated intravascular coagulation (DIC), and heparin-induced thrombocytopenia (HIT) are three such examples and will be discussed here.

Thrombocytes are cells in the blood that help with the clotting process that achieves hemostasis. A lack of thrombocytes is called a thrombocytopenia. ITP, then, is a type of thrombocytopenia that occurs in the absence of systemic disease, marked by bleeding, and often has no known cause, hence the idiopathy.

ITP is a chronic condition in adults, but usually resolves spontaneously in children. Typically the patient will present with petechiae, purpura, and mucosal bleeding. **Petechiae** are small red or purple spots that appear on the skin and mark small points of bleeding in the capillary beds. **Purpura** are a slightly larger point of collected blood under the skin that indicate uncontrolled bleeding in the capillary beds. **Ecchymosis**, or bruising, which is the largest of the bleeding lesions, may also be present in ITP.

Diagnosis of ITP is made via blood tests, with other causes of thrombocytopenia excluded to confirm diagnosis. Corticosteroids will be used to try and stop bleeding. In very severe cases of ITP, a splenectomy, in which the spleen is removed, is considered to resolve ITP. In the case of severe, uncontrolled bleeding, the patient may be given a platelet transfusion.

DIC is a medical emergency in which the coagulation cascade has been activated by exposure to a tissue factor. The fibrinolytic pathway is also activated. Usually onset of DIC is rapid, with bleeding and occlusion of the small blood vessels present. The result of a sudden onset of DIC is thrombocytopenia, a prolonged PT and PTT time, high d-Dimer, and lowered plasma fibrinogen.

Causes of DIC can include obstetric complications such as abruptio placentae, retained dead fetus, or amniotic fluid embolism. Infections with gram-negative organs that release an endotoxin that causes tissue factor release may cause DIC. Cancers usually produce a slow-onset DIC in which more clotting activities are part of the clinical presentation.

Treatment of DIC will include replacement therapy of platelets, cryoprecipitate, and fresh frozen plasma. In patients with a slower onset of DIC, heparin may be used to treat the condition.

HIT is a condition in patients receiving heparin therapy in which platelet aggregation occurs in excessive amounts leading to blockage of blood vessels. These vessel obstructions may lead to other life-threatening events such as stroke, acute MI, and occlusion of arm or leg arteries. If HIT is suspected, heparin therapy should be stopped immediately. Alternative anticoagulants such as argatroban, bivalirudin, and fondaparinux will be used until platelet count has returned to normal.

Immune Deficiencies

The immune system of the body works to fight against disease. The components of the blood that form the body's primary immune system are the white blood cells. Monocytes, lymphocytes, neutrophils, basophils, and eosinophils compose the white blood cells. Monocytes help to break down bacteria. Lymphocytes are responsible for antibody creation in the defense against invasive organisms. Neutrophils take out bacterial and fungal organisms and are the numerous first line of defense against infections. Basophils secrete histamine, the substance responsible for itching associated with allergic diseases. Eosinophils target parasites and cancer cells, and are part of the body's allergic response.

There are numerous ways the immune system can malfunction, categorized into primary and secondary causes. Primary immunodeficiency begins at birth and is inherited. Secondary conditions are acquired later in life, an example of which would be the acquisition of human immunodeficiency virus (HIV).

Primary immunodeficiencies can be further subcategorized by which part of the immunity they affect, whether that be B cells, T cells, both B and T cells, phagocytes, and/or complement proteins. In all of these subcategories, the component of the immune system affected has been reduced in number, is malfunctioning, or missing altogether, resulting in compromised immune function and disease states.

Secondary immunodeficiency can arise as a result of drug abuse or side effects of medications, chronic diabetes, or cancer. All of these predisposing factors can have long-term weakening effects on the immune system.

Examples of drugs that can weaken the immune system include corticosteroids and immunosuppressants. Corticosteroids may be used to treat inflammatory conditions, such as rheumatoid arthritis. Immunosuppressants are given to those who have recently received a tissue or organ transplant, to prevent their body from rejecting the tissue.

As a person ages, the immune system naturally weakens over time, leaving the elderly person vulnerable to infectious organisms. A condition that goes hand in hand with aging is undernutrition. As people age, their social situations may change, such with death of a spouse or close friends. These social changes, as well as a deteriorating body, may lead them to stop cooking for themselves and care less about nutrition, leading to undernutrition. Undernutrition then leads to further weakening of the immune system. Zinc deficiency and calcium deficiency are common signs of undernutrition in elderly persons.

Chronic, back to back infections is a sign of a weakened immune system. The person may present with fever, chills, weight loss, abdominal pain, or what is called "failure to thrive," meaning they are not growing and developing as normal. However, this term is commonly used for infants, rather than adults.

Prevention is the best means for handling immune deficiency. Promoting strong immune health will help fight off infections. Vaccination against diseases is helpful. Treatment of the infections with antibiotics, antifungals, and antivirals is commonplace. In some patients stem cell transplantation and immune globulin may be used in the treatment of immunodeficiency.

Leukopenia

When the white blood cells drop to a count of less than four thousand cells per microliter of blood, it is termed **leukopenia**. A person experiencing leukopenia will be more susceptible to invasive organisms and, as a result, infections, because their normal defenses are compromised. The term leukopenia may sometimes be used interchangeably with the term neutropenia. **Neutropenia** refers to a drop in the number of circulating neutrophils within the blood. Neutrophils are the most numerous component of the white blood cells; thus leukopenia and neutropenia are very similar in concept.

There are numerous causes of leukopenia within the body. A severe infection may lower the count of white blood cells, as can the side effects or abuse of certain drugs. Patients with cancers involving malignant tumors that destroy the immune system will show a lowered white blood cell count and thus be leukopenic. An enlarged spleen, termed splenomegaly or hypersplenism, may cause leukopenia.

Diagnosis of leukopenia or neutropenia will be made based upon clinical presentation of the patient and blood test measuring the count of the white blood cells. Treatment will be aimed at the underlying cause, be it infection, malignancy, or otherwise. Antimicrobial therapy may be used to target a systemic infection causing the leukopenia.

Thrombocytopenia

In the blood, there are cells called thrombocytes that play a key role in clotting, as previously mentioned. Literally meaning "blood clot cell," a thrombocyte can also be called a platelet. Thrombocytes arise from the bone marrow and are shed off of a cell called a megakaryocyte. Thrombocytes are irregularly shaped, making them excellent at clumping together and assisting with the formation of clots.

When the number of thrombocytes is lowered in the blood, a condition called thrombocytopenia occurs. This condition puts patients at increased risk for bleeding as they do not have an essential component of clotting present in adequate numbers.

There are a number of different ways thrombocytopenia can occur, arising from numerous different causes. Two main categories of thrombocytopenia are those that occur as a result of immunologic causes and those that occur as a result of nonimmunologic causes. An immunologic cause of thrombocytopenia could include a viral infection, side effects of drugs, blood transfusions, or connective tissue disorders. Nonimmunologic causes include sepsis or acute respiratory distress syndrome.

A normal count of thrombocytes or platelets is 140,000 to 440,000, though that number can vary in the case of pregnant women or persons with inflammatory conditions. A significant drop below that number is considered thrombocytopenia.

A patient with thrombocytopenia will likely exhibit signs of bleeding, the classic signs being petechiae, purpura, and ecchymoses scattered across the body. Bleeding from the mucosal regions of the body, such as the mouth, is common.

Based on clinical observations of the above signs and symptoms, as well as the patient's history and laboratory findings, diagnosis will be made. The treatment will be based on the underlying cause.

Gastrointestinal

The abdomen holds within its walls almost all the vital organs of the body, save the heart, lungs, and brain. These organs are prone to injury and disease, with one organ's ailment occasionally affecting nearby organs. The following will be a discussion of injuries and diseases affecting the abdominal region of the body, as well as the processes of the gastrointestinal tract.

Acute Abdominal Trauma

When an injury occurs that affects the abdomen, it is called an abdominal trauma. Since there are a vast number of ways in which the abdomen can be traumatized, it is helpful for the practitioner to categorize the injury. One method of categorizing abdominal trauma is by the area of the abdomen affected: the abdominal wall, one of the major solid organs, one of the hollow organs, or the vasculature of the abdomen. Examples of solid organs include the liver, spleen, pancreas, and kidneys. The hollow organs are the stomach, small intestine, colon, ureters, and bladder. The abdominal aorta would be the most serious component of the vasculature to be injured, as it carries the majority of the blood pumped out of the heart to supply the lower half of the body.

A trauma to the abdomen can be blunt or penetrating. A blow such as a kick, a fall down a set of stairs, or hitting the steering wheel in a car accident are all examples of blunt force trauma. A penetrating wound, such as a gunshot or stab wound, is one in which the abdominal wall is penetrated.

An abdominal trauma may also affect the structures surrounding it, such as the spinal cord, the vertebrae, or the pelvis.

The common manifestations of abdominal trauma are lacerations, hemorrhage, hematoma, and perforation of the contents of the abdomen, depending on where the injury occurs and the severity of the force. When a hollow viscus such as the stomach or the colon are perforated, their contents seep out into the peritoneal cavity, causing acute peritonitis.

A patient who has suffered an abdominal trauma may develop delayed complications such as rupture of a hematoma, development of an intra-abdominal abscess, an obstruction or ileus within the bowel, a leakage of bile, or compartment syndrome of the bowel.

The chief complaint of those who have abdominal injuries is abdominal pain. Blood in the urine, radiating pain to the left shoulder indicating splenic injury, and signs of hypovolemia are all indicative of abdominal injury. Tachycardia, low blood pressure, diaphoresis, pallor or duskiness, as well as altered level of consciousness are all signs that an abdominal trauma has occurred.

Depending on the injuries incurred and the severity of the patient's condition, emergency laparotomy to repair damage and stop bleeding may be necessary. In other cases, however, the patient may simply be put under observation and visual imaging tests run to determine damage and treatment plan.

Acute GI Hemorrhage

Bleeding along the gastrointestinal (GI) tract can be insidious or acute in onset, occurring anywhere along the tract from the mouth to the anus. Acute GI bleeding is more serious in nature and needs to be addressed sooner in order to prevent hypovolemic shock.

A patient experiencing an acute GI hemorrhage will present differently based on the origin of the bleed. If it is an upper GI bleed, hematemesis or bloody vomit will appear with either a coffee ground (older blood) or bright red (new blood) appearance. Bleeding originating in the lower GI tract will appear in fecal matter as black or tarry stool (old blood), dark blood, or bright red blood. It is important to note that bright red blood in the stool is sometimes a result of hemorrhoids, not a GI hemorrhage.

The hemorrhage itself is not a disease but rather a sign of underlying disease, which will determine the target of treatment. Peptic ulcers, tears in the esophagus, diverticulitis, or cancers of the GI tract are all possible culprits of an acute GI bleed.

In order to target the source of the bleed, a tool called an endoscope will often be used. Depending on the suspected region of the GI tract, whether upper or lower, an upper endoscopy or lower endoscopy may be used. Colonoscopy is the term used to refer to a scope of the colon, part of the lower GI tract. Esophagogastroduodenoscopy or EGD is a long and medically accurate way to say an endoscopy that looks at the esophagus, stomach, and duodenum.

In endoscopy, a thin tube with a camera affixed to the end of it is threaded into the body and images are produced. During endoscopy, areas that are bleeding may be cauterized to stop bleeding. **Cauterization** is the application of heat to the lesion to bring about hemostasis.

Bowel Infarction/Obstruction/Perforation

Almost one-quarter of the blood that is pumped out of the heart with each beat is required to supply the mucosa of the intestine with oxygen and other nutrients required for the metabolic activity that takes place there. An interruption to this blood flow, therefore, could lead to profound consequences. Ischemia, as discussed in the cardiac section, describes such an interruption of blood flow to tissue, which, over time, will lead to tissue death.

Acute mesenteric ischemia describes an ischemic condition of the bowel in which blood flow has been interrupted. This is a medical emergency that leads to inflammation and, eventually, infarction. **Infarction** describes total tissue death. The interruption in acute mesenteric ischemia is often caused by a blood clot. It may also be caused by a state of low blood flow, such as hypotension caused by shock.

The patient with acute mesenteric ischemia will often complain of abdominal pain. An exploratory laparotomy or angiography will be necessary to diagnose this condition. Once diagnosed, the patient may be treated by an embolectomy, in which the clot is removed. Other treatment options include resection of the bowel, in which the affected region is removed and the remaining segments reattached. Vasodilators and revascularization therapies will also be used when appropriate. This condition has a high mortality rate.

Within the bowels, obstructions may occur, causing cramping, vomiting, constipation, and decreased flatulence leading to bloating. An obstruction may be complete or partial. Diagnosis of intestinal obstruction is made by X-ray images of the abdomen as well as clinical presentation. A patient with an abdominal obstruction will be treated using fluid resuscitation, suction via nasogastric tube or, in severe cases, surgery to remove the obstruction.

The most common causes of mechanical obstruction in the bowel are adhesions, hernias, or cancerous tumors. Gallstones, diverticulitis, twisting of the bowel or volvulus, intussusception, and fecal impaction are also potential causes of obstruction.

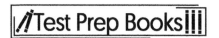

Adhesions are bands of sticky, fibrous tissue within the bowel that cause surrounding tissues and organs to stick together, resulting in obstruction and ischemic conditions of the bowel. An adhesion must be removed surgically.

Illustration of an Adhesion

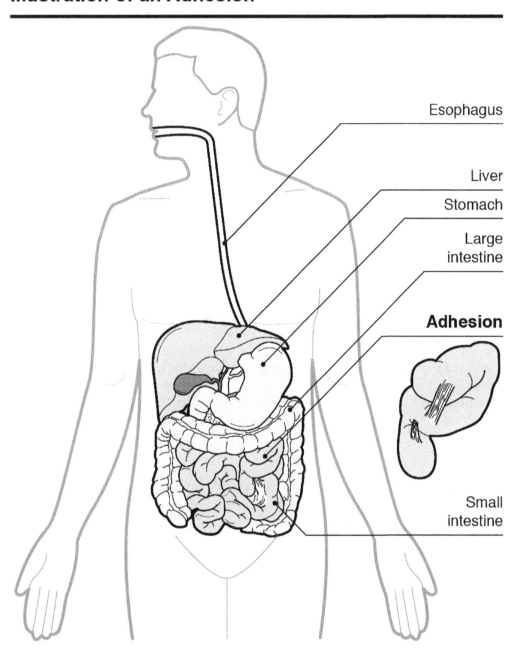

A gastrointestinal perforation refers to a hole or tear that has formed through the entire wall of an intestine, whether small or large. Symptoms of this condition include abdominal pain, vomiting, and fever. The hole must be surgically repaired and is an emergency situation. Contents of the bowel may leak out when perforation has occurred resulting in an inflammatory condition called peritonitis.

Gastroesophageal Reflux

The lower esophagus is sealed off from the acidic environment of the stomach by way of a muscular sphincter. When this sphincter weakens and contents of the stomach leak up into the esophagus, it is called gastroesophageal reflux disease (GERD). The burning sensation caused by stomach acid coming in contact with the lining of the lower esophagus is the tell-tale sign of GERD.

Risk factors for the development of GERD include weight gain, cigarette smoking, and drug side effects. Antihistamines, tricyclic antidepressants, nitrates, and calcium channel blockers are all examples of drugs that may contribute to the development of GERD.

A patient will be diagnosed with GERD based on symptomology, with the occasional endoscopy used to confirm the diagnosis. The patient will be encouraged to make diet changes, be prescribed proton pump inhibitors and, in very severe cases, surgical repair may be recommended.

Diet changes will include avoiding consuming substances that aggravate the condition such as coffee, alcohol, and fatty foods. Smoking cessation will be encouraged as this also can be an aggravating factor.

Omeprazole is a commonly prescribed proton pump inhibitor used in the treatment of GERD, along with lansoprazole, pantoprazole, and esomeprazole.

Long-standing GERD may lead to further complications, such as esophagitis, peptic esophageal ulcer, esophageal stricture, Barrett esophagus, and even cancerous tumors of the esophagus.

GI Surgeries

There are many conditions of the various organs of the abdomen that may need surgical intervention to fix.

A cholecystectomy is a procedure in which the entire gallbladder is removed. The gallbladder is a pear-shaped organ that is positioned below the liver and adjacent to the stomach. The decision to take out the gallbladder is based on patient condition and, specifically, if gallstone formation is causing pain.

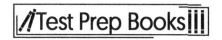

Cholecystectomy begins with the physician inflating the abdomen for a clear view with which to work. After this, the physician makes small incisions and insets a thin tube with a camera at the end into the abdomen. The physician visualizes the gallbladder and then removes it. This type of surgical procedure, in which there is minimal invasion, a camera or scope is used, and smaller incisions are made, is called a laparoscopic procedure.

Illustration showing cholecystectomy using the minimally-invasive laparoscopic procedure

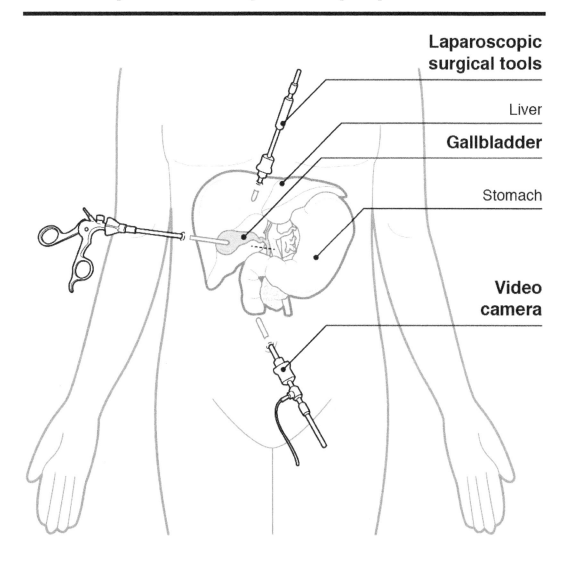

Other surgical interventions of the upper organs of the GI tract include hiatal hernia repair, removal of cancerous tumors, removal of hepatic cysts, and repair of ulcerative conditions.

Surgeries involving the lower GI tract include hemorrhoidectomy (removal of hemorrhoids), repair of anal fistulas, resection of the bowels, ileostomy, and colostomy.

Ileostomy and colostomy are surgical procedures in which a portion of the bowel is rerouted up through a hole in the abdomen. Ileostomy involves the small intestine or ileum, while colostomy involves the large intestine or colon. These two procedures are performed in the cases of severe bowel disease, such as bowel cancer, diverticulitis, and inflammatory bowel disease.

The patient with a stoma as a result of an ileostomy or colostomy will need to be educated on how to care for it. A bag is attached to the stoma for the purpose of collecting fecal matter. This bag can be taken off and replaced as needed. The stoma needs to be assessed regularly to make sure it has not become infected. The stoma should be pink, and the area surrounding it should be kept clean and dry.

Healthy stoma site postcolostomy

Stoma is pink; area surrounding is clean and dry

Stoma

Hepatic Failure/Coma

Acute hepatic failure is a condition in which the liver is no longer performing at its normal level of metabolic function. Acute hepatic failure is most often caused by drug toxicity or viral infection. For instance, the pain reliever and fever reducer acetaminophen is known to cause liver damage and failure in toxic overdoses. The common viral culprit of liver failure is hepatitis B, with hepatitis C being less common.

A patient experiencing liver failure will exhibit signs of encephalopathy—including confusion—as well as jaundice and ascites. Jaundice is a yellowing of the skin and ascites is a severe bloat of the abdomen as a result of massive collection of free fluid. In severe cases, this fluid will be drained off the abdomen to relieve pressure.

Portal hypertension is a condition most often caused by cirrhosis or scarring of the liver in which the pressure of the portal vein is elevated. The portal vein drains blood from the organs of the upper GI tract, such as the spleen, intestines, and pancreas into the liver. When the liver cannot receive the normal amount of blood due to scarring or disease, the resistance to the incoming blood rises, resulting in the higher pressure. Complications of portal hypertension include ascites, splenomegaly, and acute variceal bleeding. Variceal bleeding has a high mortality rate as it is difficult to control.

Treatment of portal hypertension includes monitoring, banding via endoscopy, and pharmacologic therapy, such as beta-blockers.

Cirrhosis is a scarring of the liver tissue over time and is an associated condition of acute liver failure. Chronic alcoholism is a leading cause of cirrhosis. The scarring of the liver can be slowed with treatment and alcohol abuse cessation, but ultimately is irreversible.

Esophageal varices are dilated veins located in the esophagus and are a result of portal hypertension. These varices are highly vulnerable to massive bleeding, but are otherwise asymptomatic. Esophageal varices may be treated with banding procedures as well as intravenous administration of octreotide.

Fulminant hepatitis is a type of acute liver failure that occurs without the presence of pre-existing, chronic disease states. This type of liver failure is usually preceded by hepatic viruses, exposure to toxins, or drug injury. Fulminant hepatitis causes a large amount of necrosis or tissue death in the liver. As a result, liver transplantation may be needed in order for the patient to fully recover.

Biliary atresia is a condition of the bile duct in which it is blocked or possibly even absent. This condition occurs in newborns because of abnormal fetal development. Newborns with biliary atresia are jaundiced because of the bile-duct atresia. A procedure called the Kasai procedure is often used to repair biliary atresia. In this procedure, the small intestine is attached to the liver to create a new pathway for bile to drain. The intestine is then reattached to a lower portion of the small intestine to reconnect it with the GI tract. Many infants with biliary atresia will develop liver failure later in life and will likely need liver transplants.

Illustration of the Kasai procedure performed for biliary atresia

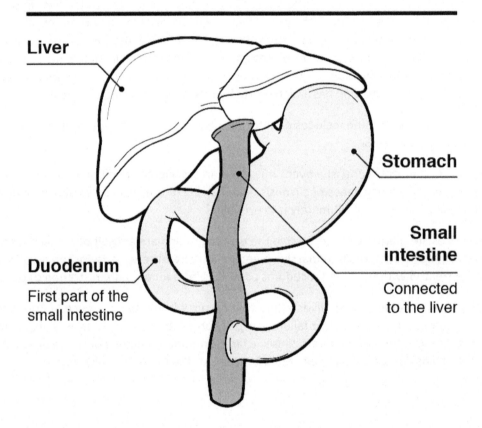

Liver

Stomach

Small intestine
Connected to the liver

Duodenum
First part of the small intestine

Malnutrition and Malabsorption

Malnutrition is a disorder that includes overnutrition and undernutrition. Overnutrition is a form of malnutrition that is associated with obesity and metabolic syndrome, in which a person is consuming far more calories from food than needed for healthy body function. Undernutrition is a result of deficient consumption of necessary nutrients for the body's function. Nutrients can be lost as a result of diarrhea or vomiting, leading to an undernourished state. Anorexia, a psychological condition in which a person refrains from eating in order to lose weight to achieve an unrealistic body image, is another form of undernutrition.

Progression of malnutrition may be slow or rapid, depending on the case. Anorexia is a slow decline in nourishment, while the body wasting or cachexia associated with cancers may result in rapid undernourishment.

Undernutrition often manifests as weakness, muscle wasting, weight loss, and irritability. The patient may become pale and fatigued.

Treatment of undernutrition includes diet control, correction of fluid and electrolyte irregularities, and correction of complications that may have developed.

Malabsorption is a disorder of the small intestine in which nutrients are not properly absorbed into the blood stream, resulting in a malnourished state of the body. Chronic diarrhea is the most common manifestation of malabsorption. **Steatorrhea**, or fatty stools, is a common sign of malabsorption, reflecting the fat loss of the body. Treatment of malabsorption will be aimed at correcting the cause. Common causes of malabsorption include bacterial overgrown syndrome, celiac disease, Whipple disease, and short-bowel syndrome.

Pancreatitis

Pancreatitis is an inflammation of the pancreas. The pancreas functions as both an exocrine and an endocrine gland. Inflammation results in a decrease in the pancreas's ability to function in these capacities. The condition can be either chronic or acute, with chronic pancreatitis leading to irreversible damage, fibrosis, and strictures of the ductal systems of the pancreas.

Major risk factors for developing chronic pancreatitis include alcohol abuse and smoking cigarettes. A patient will likely present with severe abdominal pain, centered around the epigastric region of the abdomen, that may be relieved or partially relieved by leaning forward or sitting up.

Treatment of pancreatitis will target control of the pain associated with flare-ups. Enzymes of the pancreas may be supplemented and complications such as diabetes will be managed.

Renal/Genitourinary

The kidneys are responsible for maintaining a healthy fluid and electrolyte balance in the body through filtration, reabsorption, and excretory processes. Urine is formed in the kidney, drained through the ureters to the bladder, and then excreted via urination. When these vital processes are interrupted by diseases, disorders, and injuries, imbalances occur. The following will be a discussion of diseases of the renal and genitourinary tract.

Acute Kidney Injuries (AKIs), Acute Renal Failure (ARF), and Acute Tubular Necrosis (ATN)

An acute kidney injury and acute renal failure are essentially interchangeable terms referring to a rapid decline in kidney function. The course of dysfunction may last for days to weeks, with a build-up of nitrogenous waste products in the blood stream as a result. The cause of acute injury or failure may be a severe blow, such as blunt force trauma. Illnesses and surgical procedures may also cause the kidneys to fail.

Patients experiencing AKI or ARF may present with symptoms of nausea, anorexia, and vomiting, which are all reactions to the excessive waste products polluting the body. In severe cases, the patient may experience seizures or coma. When the kidney is no longer performing at capacity, fluid, electrolyte, and acid-base imbalances will develop. AKI is treated based on cause, with fluid and electrolyte rebalance being the target. In some cases, dialysis may be necessary.

One of the most common causes of ARF is acute tubular necrosis. The tubular cells of the kidney are key to its function. They work to absorb and help filtrate vital fluid and electrolytes, as well as help form urine. When the kidney is hypoperfused or injured, such as is the case in hypotensive crises or when nephrotoxic drugs are taken, the tubular cells begin to die and kidney failure results.

Symptomology is like that of ARF and AKI, since ATN is a causative factor. Oliguria, or little to no urine production, is a sign of ATN that has developed into ARF. Correcting the cause of ATN, as well as neutralizing nephrotoxins and correcting fluid and electrolyte imbalances, will help bring the patient's kidney function back to normal.

Chronic Kidney Disease (CKD)

While acute injury and failure of the kidney can often be corrected, chronic kidney disease is a slow, progressive, and irreversible decline in function of the kidney. The most common causes of CKD are diabetes, hypertension, and diseases of the glomerulus. Metabolic syndrome, in which the patient has both diabetes and hypertension, is a major factor in CKD development.

Over time, these causative factors slowly destroy vital cells in the renal tissue. Renal function first becomes insufficient and then fails altogether, which is called end-stage renal disease (ESRD).

As the kidney fails, waste products build up in the body. Creatinine and urea are markers for kidney decline, though they are not the only waste products that cause the symptoms of uremia, or "urine in the blood." Sodium, water, potassium, and other fluid and electrolyte imbalances will occur as a result of CKD.

The kidney is responsible for releasing erythropoietin, a hormone that stimulates the production of red blood cells. When kidneys fail, as is the case in CKD, erythropoietin release is decreased as well, resulting in decreased erythropoiesis, or RBC production. Thus, anemia results. Patients with CKD often must be treated for anemia along with many other conditions.

A patient with CKD will present with weight loss, anorexia, nausea, vomiting, and stomatitis. They may have a yellow-brown tint to their skin, as well as itchiness and crystallization of their sweat called **uremic frost.**

Treating a patient with CKD is a complicated matter, as so many other systems are involved as a result of the kidneys failing. Management of diabetes and hypertension is crucial, as these are often the underlying causes. Heart failure and anemia must be addressed. Dialysis will likely be an option in the future of the CKD patient to replace the function of the kidney.

Incontinence

Incontinence refers to losing one's ability to control the bowel and bladder. Urinary incontinence will be discussed here.

There are four types of urinary incontinence: stress, functional, urge, and overflow. When urine leaks after an irrepressible urge to urinate, it is called urge incontinence. When intra-abdominal pressure increases and causes urine leakage, it is called stress incontinence. When the bladder is filled with too much urine without the urge to void and urine leaks as a result, it is called overflow incontinence. When physical or cognitive impairments cause a person to lose control of their bladder, this is called functional incontinence.

Identifying the exact cause or mechanism of urinary incontinence is key to reversing its progression. Bladder training and Kegel exercises have been shown to improve outcomes in patients with urinary incontinence. There are certain drugs that may help with urinary incontinence. Duloxetine acts to increase urinary sphincter muscle tone and may be used in cases of urinary incontinence.

Infections

Urinary tract infections or UTIs can be divided into two categories: lower and upper. Upper UTIs affect the kidneys and can be called pyelonephritis. Lower UTIs affect the bladder, urethra, or prostate and can be called cystitis, urethritis, or prostatitis. Differentiating between the specific types of UTIs in clinical practice can be difficult to do and thus the broad term of UTI usually refers to an infection of the kidneys or bladder.

There are many causative organisms involved in UTIs, but the most commonly seen UTIs are caused by a bacterial infection. Fungal infections, usually arising from the candida species, are also a possibility, as well as parasites and viruses.

An infection that affects the urethra specifically, called urethritis, is likely a result of a sexually transmitted disease (STD).

A urinary tract infection that was caught as a result of a urinary catheter insertion is called a catheter-associated urinary tract infection (CAUTI). These are of special interest to the critical care nurse as so many patients have catheters inserted while in critical care. The critical care nurse must take special care to use proper aseptic technique when inserting a catheter, remove catheters as soon as they are no longer needed, and follow facility procedure when deciding if a patient actually needs a catheter in the first place. Many patients have catheters that may not need them, setting them up for a hospital-acquired infection.

Patients who have contracted a UTI may be asymptomatic for some time before the UTI is detected. When they are symptomatic, they may present with a fever, altered mental status, hypotension, dysuria, and lower abdominal pain.

Urine will be cultured and, in the case of patients with indwelling catheters, the catheter tip will be cultured as well to obtain diagnosis of UTI. Antibiotic therapy is common in the treatment of UTI, depending on the cause.

Life-Threatening Electrolyte Imbalances

One of the kidney's most important jobs is to maintain a healthy balance of fluid and electrolytes in the body. Imbalances in these substances, such as potassium, sodium, magnesium, and calcium, can be life-threatening and need emergent medical intervention.

When potassium levels exceed normal, it is called hyperkalemia. There are different grades of hyperkalemia. An amount greater than 5.0 mEq/L is considered mildly hyperkalemic, while moderate hyperkalemia is 6.0 mEq/L to 7.0 mEq/L, and severe hyperkalemia is greater than 7.0 mEq/L. Hyperkalemia will manifest itself on the ECG as tented T waves, widening QRS waves and deep S waves. The patient may go into cardiac arrest as a result of a toxic level of potassium running through their veins. If hyperkalemia is suspected, any potassium the patient is receiving must be immediately stopped. If it is a severe case of hyperkalemia, potassium needs to be immediately shifted back into the cells using one or a combination of the following therapies: glucose plus insulin, sodium bicarbonate, calcium chloride, and/or nebulized albuterol.

Low potassium, called hypokalemia, is defined as a potassium level of less than 3.5 mEq/L. This can be caused by diarrhea or massive fluid volume loss from the kidneys. A patient with hypokalemia may exhibit weakness, polyuria, cardiac cells that are hyperexcitable, and muscle cramping. Potassium must be replaced, whether orally or via IV infusions, depending on the severity of the case. The critical care nurse must monitor for over-supplementation that turns into hyperkalemia, especially in patients with ESRD whose kidneys cannot properly metabolize and regulate potassium.

Integumentary

The largest organ of the body is the skin, protecting the internal environment of the body from the external environment. To prevent infections and promote healing, the critical care nurse needs to be knowledgeable about the conditions that compromise the skin's integrity.

IV Infiltration

Most patients the critical care nurse will care for in the critical care unit will require an IV infusion of some kind. A complication of peripheral IV therapy that the nurse must be watchful for is IV infiltration. An infiltration of an IV means that the IV catheter has become dislodged or misplaced within the tissue and IV fluid or medications are leaking into the surrounding tissue as a result. This also can be caused by a sudden movement or jerking motion by the patient.

Patients with an altered mental status are prone to IV infiltration due to their at times compulsive, uncontrolled movements. This behavior can lead to dislodgment of the IV catheter and result in IV infiltration.

When an IV has infiltrated, the tissue surrounding the site may become puffy, tight, cool, and swollen. The patient, if alert, may complain of discomfort and burning. The IV pump infusing the fluids or medications may begin to beep and normal interventions may do nothing to help, thus infiltration should always be suspected.

Some fluids and medications can be toxic to the tissues and must be carefully monitored for infiltrations. An example of this is toxic chemotherapy drugs, which are often infused through a centralized port for just this reason.

Prevention of IV infiltration includes proper IV placement technique, educating the patient on signs of infiltration, and frequent monitoring and assessment of the IV sites. Most IVs and dressings must be changed frequently to prevent infiltration, and the critical care nurse must follow related facility policies.

Pressure Ulcers

Most critical care nurses that have had to deal with immobile, bedridden patients who are very ill are familiar with pressure ulcers. Because of immobility, pressure against vulnerable parts of the body results in tissue necrosis and ulceration. Bony prominences are especially susceptible to ulceration.

Risk factors for developing pressure ulcers include increased age, immobility, undernutrition, and urinary and/or fecal incontinence. Factors that contribute to pressure ulcers include shear, friction, pressure, and moisture. Increased exposure in compromised patients results in ulcerization.

Ulcers can be staged into several categories, including stages I, II, III, and IV, unstageable, and suspected deep tissue injury (DTI). Each category looks at depth of wound and tissues affected. Wounds do not necessarily progress from one stage to the next; they can sometimes develop very quickly, skipping stages.

Prevention is obviously the best intervention when addressing pressure ulcers. The critical care nurse can help prevent pressure ulcers by turning the patient every two hours, reducing pressure where possible with pillows and supports, encouraging early mobilization and proper nutrition, and meticulously caring for wounds that do develop to prevent infection and loss of tissue.

Wounds

Knowing how to care for each wound type is crucial to restoring the patient back to their normal functioning ability. There are three distinct types of wounds that a critical care nurse may encounter in their practice: infectious, surgical, and traumatic:

Infectious

A wound that has become infected is called an infectious wound. This means that bacteria and other microorganisms have invaded and colonized. This infection can delay healing and spread to other tissues of the body or even to the body's internal system. Any wound a patient develops, whether a pressure ulcer, trauma wound, or surgical wound, may become infected, thus the critical care nurse must be aware of signs and symptoms.

An infectious wound may become reddened or painful, swell as a result of inflammation, discharge a pus-like fluid that is green or yellow, be malodorous, and not heal as a result of the infection.

Staphylococcus aureus is a common bacterial invader of wounds, as it is often found on normal skin. The wound is its entryway to becoming a full-blown infection.

Those at risk for developing infectious wounds are the elderly, diabetics, and those who are immunocompromised, such as patients with the HIV infection.

Surgical

A surgical wound is a natural byproduct of any surgery. Whether a small or large incision, the surgeon has to open the body cavity in some way, shape, or form to access the internal tissue or organ he/she needs to operate on. Surgical wounds will usually be dressed by the operating room (OR) team, but the critical care nurse will be in charge of monitoring the wound and changing the dressing while the patient is in the critical care unit. A surgical wound will often have **sutures**, or tiny stitches that are sewn onto the patient's skin, in place. Sometimes these sutures will dissolve and be absorbed by the patient and sometimes they will need to be removed after a certain amount of time, depending on the procedure, the surgeon, and the facility policy on the subject.

The signs of a surgical wound that has become infected are the same as any infectious wound: redness, swelling, discharge of pus, odor, pain, and lack of healing.

Trauma

A trauma wound differs from a surgical wound in that its openings will usually be irregular and large. Bleeding is a major factor in traumatic wounds due to their depth and size. Bleeding must be stopped and the wound must be closed before any dressing may be placed and healing can begin. Typically, this will be handled in the emergency department or the surgical suite, but the critical care nurse receiving the patient in the critical care unit will be responsible for further monitoring of the wound, dressing changes, and assessing for healing.

Most dressing changes are recommended daily, usually to be administered with an antibiotic cream. Dressing changes may be more or less frequent depending on the wound and the surgeon's orders. The critical care nurse will follow suit.

Practice Questions

1. A patient who has been NPO (nothing by mouth) all morning for a cardiac catheterization complains of nausea and "just not feeling right." The nurse notices that he is sweating. What condition should the nurse suspect and investigate right away?
   a. Hypochondria
   b. Hypoglycemia *sweating, nausea, malaise → po glucagon*
   c. Hypotension
   d. Hypothyroidism

X 2. A decreased amount of vasopressin in the body will likely produce which of the following conditions?
   a. SIADH
   b. Diabetes type I *polyuria*   *↑ Ø enough anti - diuretic - hormone*
   c. Diabetes insipidus *decreased vasopressin from pituitary = massive diuresis/hypovolemia*
   d. Diabetes type II *polyuria*

X 3. Which of the following metabolic components involved in diabetic ketoacidosis is responsible for the "fruity" smell that a person with DKA gives off when they breathe?
   a. Alanine *fat/muscle breakdown*
   b. Triglycerides
   c. Acetone *ketoacid produced by breakdown of fatty acids*
   d. Glycerol *fat/muscle breakdown*

4. High blood sugar stimulates the kidneys to do which of the following?
   a. Produce less urine
   b. Concentrate the urine
   c. Retain more sodium
   d. Produce more urine

5. Which body system will exhibit the most obvious effects of a state of hyperosmolar hyperglycemic nonketotic syndrome (HHNK)?
   a. Neurologic
   b. Cardiac
   c. Endocrine
   d. Pulmonary

X 6. To correct the hyponatremia associated with syndrome of inappropriate antidiuretic hormone, which of the following solutions is used?
   a. Normal saline
   b. Hypertonic saline *concentrated, helps correct unconcentrated blood*
   c. Hypotonic saline
   d. Lactated ringer's solution

79

7. Which of the following anemia categories, in which heme and globin do not synthesize appropriately, does thalassemia fall into?
    a. Thrombocytic =platelets
    b. Macrocytic large, oddly shaped, compromising o2 carry capacity
    c. Normocytic normal cells, defecient in #
    d. Microcytic

8. Where should nurses assess for pallor in a patient with dark skin who is suspected to be anemic?
    a. Forearms
    b. Cheeks
    c. Conjunctiva w/ palms, bottom of feet, bucal mucosa
    d. Scalp

9. A patient with idiopathic thrombocytopenia purpura presents with the classic purpura on the skin. Which of the following statements explains how to differentiate between the signs and symptoms of a thrombocytopenia?
    a. Purpura are larger than petechiae, but smaller than ecchymoses
    b. Purpura are larger than both petechiae and ecchymoses
    c. Purpura are smaller than both petechiae and ecchymoses
    d. Purpura are smaller than petechiae, but larger than ecchymoses

10. A patient experiencing itching related to an allergic reaction likely has the substance histamine being secreted by which white blood cell?
    a. Eosinophils
    b. Basophils secrete histamine
    c. Neutrophils take out infection
    d. Monocytes break down bacteria

11. Which term is used interchangeably with leukopenia, a condition in which the white blood cell count is lower than normal?
    a. Thrombocytopenia
    b. Lymphocytopenia
    c. Neutropenia
    d. Monocytopenia

12. Which of the following causes of thrombocytopenia is considered an immunological cause?
    a. Folate deficiency
    b. Drug side effects
    c. Acute respiratory distress syndrome
    d. Viral infection

13. A twenty-two-year-old male comes in with a gunshot wound to the right upper quadrant of his abdomen. The bleeding has been controlled, the wound was closed, and he has been hemodynamically stabilized. What solid organ of the abdomen does the nurse suspect might have been hit by the gunshot?
    a. Stomach
    b. Small intestine
    c. Liver
    d. Colon

14. A thirty-three-year-old female presents to the emergency room complaining of vomiting blood. Which description of the hematemesis indicates an active upper GI bleed?
    a. Coffee ground
    b. Bright red
    c. Large amount
    d. Small amount

15. A fifty-five-year-old male is undergoing an endoscopy to discover the source of his hematemesis. The gastroenterologist encounters an active, bleeding lesion. What procedure using the application of heat to seal the lesion will probably be used next?
    a. Banding
    b. Biopsy
    c. Angioplasty
    d. Cauterization

16. A fifty-two-year-old male presents to the ED complaining of burning in his chest. He is a long-time pack-a-day smoker, suffers from hypertension, and is overweight. What diagnosis does the nurse suspect?
    a. CAD
    b. TIA
    c. GERD
    d. MI

17. A sixty-eight-year-old woman with a history of gallstones is in the same-day surgery unit today for a cholecystectomy. This procedure will likely be performed using which technique that involves small incisions and minimal invasion?
    a. Laparoscopic
    b. Endoscopic
    c. Bronchoscopic
    d. Laparotomy

18. A sixty-year-old male with a history of alcohol abuse and IV drug abuse presents to the emergency department with encephalopathy, ascites, and jaundice. Which organ of the abdomen does the nurse suspect is in failure?
    a. Kidney
    b. Liver
    c. Stomach
    d. Spleen

19. The nurse has a sixteen-year-old girl as a patient who is pale, fatigued, underweight, and refusing to eat, with a history of psychological issues. With what diagnosis will this girl likely be admitted to the hospital?
    a. Overnutrition
    b. Malabsorption
    c. Gastritis
    d. Anorexia

20. A 52-year-old male is admitted with symptoms of severe abdominal pain centered around the epigastric region of the abdomen and has a history of alcohol abuse and cigarette smoking. The nurse suspects which of the following conditions will be diagnosed?
    a. Gastritis
    b. Hepatitis
    c. Pancreatitis abd pain w/ hx
    d. Kidney failure

21. A thirty-nine-year-old female has been admitted with acute tubular necrosis (ATN) and is receiving IV medications to rebalance fluid and electrolyte abnormalities. Which of the following precipitating events likely led to her developing kidney failure?
    a. Hypertensive crisis
    b. Acetaminophen overdose
    c. Upper respiratory tract infection
    d. Hypotensive crisis

22. Which side effect of chronic kidney disease indicates a decrease in the release of erythropoietin?
    a. Anemia
    b. Leukemia
    c. Hypovolemia
    d. Hypocalcemia

23. A seventy-three-year-old male has developed urinary incontinence related to cognitive impairments as a result of a stroke. Which of the following drugs may be prescribed to increase urinary sphincter tone and prevent incontinence?
    a. Furosemide
    b. Duloxetine
    c. Doxazosin
    d. Finasteride

24. Which technique is most appropriate when inserting a urinary catheter into a patient to help in the prevention of CAUTIs?
    a. Sterile
    b. Clean
    c. Sanitary
    d. Aseptic

25. The nurse is looking at a patient's ECG and notices tented T waves, a widening QRS wave, and deepened S waves. She suspects which life-threatening imbalance is occurring?
    a. Hyperkalemia
    b. Hypernatremia
    c. Hypokalemia
    d. Hyponatremia

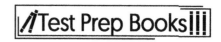

26. The nurse notices the site around the patient's peripheral IV has become puffy, cold, and tight. She suspects what has occurred?
    a. Infection
    b. IV infiltration
    c. Allergic reaction
    d. Nothing, this is a normal assessment of peripheral IV

27. Which of the following interventions will not help prevent a pressure ulcer from occurring in a bedridden patient?
    a. Turning the patient every two hours
    b. Encouraging early mobility
    c. Removing the pillows from the bed
    d. Proper nutrition

28. When assessing a patient's wound, reddening, malodor, and pus discharge are sign of what?
    a. Healing
    b. Surgery
    c. Trauma
    d. Infection

29. A twenty-nine-year-old patient has undergone a C-section and has returned to the unit. The nurse knows that he will oversee all of the following except which duty?
    a. Maintaining a clean dressing daily
    b. Monitoring for infection
    c. Applying prescribed medications
    d. Re-suturing if the incision opens

30. An eighteen-year-old female comes in with a gunshot wound to the abdomen. Which of the following takes highest priority when caring for this patient?
    a. Fluid resuscitation
    b. Stopping the bleeding
    c. Monitoring for infection
    d. Assessing internal damage

Answer Explanations

1. B: The nurse should suspect hypoglycemia based on the circumstances and symptoms being experienced by the patient. Hypoglycemia may occur when a patient receiving insulin therapy, as may be the case here if the patient is diabetic, has been NPO for a procedure. Fasting in addition to insulin therapy, if not carefully monitored and tweaked, will likely cause hypoglycemia. Sweating, nausea, and malaise are all hypoglycemic symptoms. A blood sugar reading should be immediately obtained to determine if hypoglycemia is the cause and, if so, treated with oral glucagon. Hypochondria is always possible but should be a diagnosis made by a psychiatrist. Hypotension is a less likely option given the circumstances, though not completely improbable. Hypothyroidism is unlikely and not a condition that the nurse would be able to independently diagnose without proper lab work and clinical workup.

2. C: Diabetes insipidus is caused by a decreased amount of vasopressin secreted by the pituitary gland in the body. This decrease will cause massive diuresis, leading to dehydration and hypovolemia. SIADH is the opposite situation in which vasopressin is overly released, also called antidiuretic hormone, and fluid is retained, leading to hyponatremia. Diabetes type I and diabetes type II, the two types of diabetes mellitus, share the name diabetes but are slightly different. Diabetes describes a condition in which polyuria occurs, and in the case of diabetes mellitus (mellitus is Greek for *like honey*, describing the sweetness of urine in diabetes mellitus), it is because of hyperglycemia that the polyuria occurs.

3. C: Acetone, a ketoacid produced during the breakdown of fatty acids during diabetic ketoacidosis, is expelled through respiration, thus giving a person in DKA a "fruity" smell to the breath. Glycerol and alanine are byproducts of fat and muscle breakdown as alternative energy sources convert to glucose. Triglycerides are broken down into free fatty acids as another alternative to glucose as energy for metabolism in the body.

4. D: Massive urine production, or polyuria, is the result of a hyperglycemic state in the body and a hallmark sign of any diabetic condition. Urine is not concentrated, but rather diluted. Sodium, potassium, and other electrolyte imbalances may occur as a result of polyuria, but are not a direct effect of hyperglycemia.

5. A: The most obvious effects of the super-concentrated blood that are characteristic of HHNK will appear neurologically. Confusion, seizures, coma, stroke-like syndromes, dizziness, and drowsiness are all neurological symptoms that appear in HHNK. The other systems of the body, such as cardiac, endocrine, and pulmonary may be affected but are not directly associated with the usual symptomology of HHNK.

6. B: Hypertonic saline, in which the sodium is more concentrated, is often used to correct the dilutional hyponatremia of SIADH. Normal saline has a 0.9% concentration of sodium, which is the same as circulating blood and thus will not be helpful in correcting hyponatremia. Hypotonic saline, in which there is less than 0.9% concentration of sodium, will also not be helpful in restoring normal sodium levels to the blood. Lactated ringer's solution is not a fluid used for the purpose of restoring normal sodium levels.

7. D: Thalassemia is considered a microcytic anemia, in which heme and globin do not synthesize appropriately and oxygen-carrying capacity is compromised. Normocytic anemias are those that include normally sized red blood cells that are deficient in number. Aplastic anemia is an example of a normocytic anemia. Macrocytic anemias are defined as red blood cells that are quite large in shape,

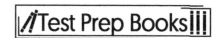

leading to abnormalities in oxygen-carrying ability and oxygen delivery. Thrombocytic refers to a platelet, a different component of the blood, and is thus irrelevant in this scenario.

8. C: A person with dark skin tones who is suspected to be anemic will show pallor in the conjunctiva of the eyes, along with the palms of the hands, bottoms of feet, buccal mucosa, and lips. Forearms, scalp, and cheeks will not show pallor, per se, but may show a gray, ashy hue if they are truly anemic.

9. A: It is true that purpura are larger than petechiae and smaller than ecchymoses or bruises. Bruises are the largest lesion of thrombocytopenia, characterized by a large pooling of blood beneath the skin. Petechiae are the smallest lesion of thrombocytopenia, characterized as tiny, pinpoint, red, flat dots on the skin. Purpura fall between ecchymoses and petechiae in size.

10. B: Basophils are the white blood cells that secrete histamine, the substance that causes itching in allergic reactions. Lymphocytes are responsible for antibody creation. Neutrophils take out bacterial and fungal organisms and are quite numerous. Monocytes assist in breaking down bacterial organisms.

11. C. Neutrophils are the most numerous of the white blood cells, which is the reason why the general term leukopenia is often used interchangeably with the slightly more specific term neutropenia. Monocytopenia and lymphocytopenia both refer to lower than normal levels of two other types of white blood cells. Thrombocytopenia is unrelated to the white blood cells, but rather refers to a lowered platelet count, a different component of the blood.

12. D: There are two categories of causes for thrombocytopenia: immunologic and nonimmunologic. A viral infection is considered an immunologic cause as the immune system is weakened by the viral infection and thrombocyte levels drop as a result. Nonimmunological causes arise from a source outside of the immune system, such as sepsis and acute respiratory distress syndrome. Folate deficiency is unrelated to thrombocytopenia but rather a cause for anemia.

13. C: The liver is a solid organ located in the right upper quadrant of the abdomen. When a penetrating wound such as a gunshot has occurred to the abdomen, it is important to be mindful of organ damage underneath the point of penetration. The small intestine, stomach, and colon are all hollow organs located in different areas of the abdomen.

14. B: Bright red blood that is being vomited usually indicates an active upper GI bleed. Coffee ground blood indicates the blood has been sitting in the stomach for a while, indicating a slower bleed. The amount of blood, whether large or small, does not indicate active bleeding necessarily. It could be a small amount vomited, but a large bleed that has not fully manifested itself.

15. D: The gastroenterologist will likely use cauterization, an application of heat, to seal the bleeding lesion. Banding is a procedure used to help stop bleeding in esophageal varices. Biopsy is where tissues are removed for histological analysis. Angioplasty is performed in cardiac catheterizations and involves balloon inflation and stent placement to open up occluded blood vessels.

16. C: The nurse suspects a diagnosis of gastroesophageal reflux disease based on the burning sensation the patient complains of and the risk factors he has (hypertension, obesity, and cigarette smoking). A myocardial infarction (MI) can sometimes be confused with GERD in symptomology as the heart and esophagus are in close proximity to each other. However, an MI usually presents as a heavy, crushing weight rather than a burning sensation. Coronary artery disease (CAD) usually is found after the patient has had an MI and involves blockages in the coronary arteries caused by atherosclerosis. Transient ischemic attack would present with stroke-like symptoms, not a burning sensation in the chest.

17. A: A laparoscopic procedure is minimally invasive and makes very small incisions for the surgeon to enter the abdominal cavity and remove the gall bladder. Laparotomy involves the surgeon making a large incision to completely open up the abdominal cavity. Endoscopy is a general term referring to an interior examination of the body—usually an examination of the upper GI tract. Bronchoscopy is one type of endoscopy that nonsurgically examines the airways and lungs.

18. B: The patient is in hepatic (liver) failure based on the symptomology and the presentation. Kidney failure would present with electrolyte and fluid abnormalities and their symptoms. Diseases of the stomach would present with GI symptoms such as nausea, vomiting, and abdominal pain in the left upper quadrant. Diseases of the spleen would manifest as blood disorders and would not be similar to symptoms of liver failure.

19. D: The patient appears to be anorexic, a psychological condition in which a patient is undernourished as a result of refusing to eat in order to meet some "ideal image" of body weight that is unrealistic. A patient with anorexia will appear pale, fatigued, underweight, and very thin. Gastritis is an inflammation of the lining of the stomach that would cause nausea, vomiting, and loss of appetite but is not applicable here. Overnutrition is a type of malnutrition associated with obesity and weight gain, not weight loss. Malabsorption is a type of nutritive disorder in which the small intestine does not absorb nutrients from food properly. Malabsorption could definitely lead to weight loss and the other symptoms but the patient's psychological issues and refusal to eat suggest a psychological condition rather than a physical disorder.

20. C: Pancreatitis is the likely diagnosis based on the location of the abdominal pain and the patient's history. The hallmark symptom of pancreatitis is abdominal pain, and that is the focus of treatment. Hepatitis presents with symptoms of liver dysfunction such as jaundice, ascites, enlargement of liver, and encephalopathy. Gastritis, an inflammation of the lining of the stomach, will present with nausea and vomiting. Kidney failure will present with oliguria and fluid and electrolyte imbalances.

21. D: A hypotensive crisis could definitely lead to necrosis of the tubular cells of the kidney due to lack of perfusion. Hypoperfusion can lead to kidney failure. A hypertensive crisis would not have the same effect on the kidney cells, though hypertension over the long term can cause kidney damage. An upper respiratory infection would likely have no effect on the kidneys. Acetaminophen overdose would affect the liver, as it is metabolized there and not in the kidneys. Nephrotoxic drugs include ibuprofen and are damaging to the kidneys in high doses.

22. A: Anemia, or a lack of red blood cells, in a patient with chronic kidney disease could indicate that erythropoietin release is decreased, meaning erythropoiesis is not being stimulated. Leukemia is a lack of white blood cells that is not affected by kidney failure. Hypovolemia is not related to a lack of erythropoietin. Hypocalcemia is an electrolyte abnormality affected by kidney failure but not by lack of erythropoietin.

23. B: Duloxetine may be prescribed for urinary incontinence to help increase sphincter muscle tone. Furosemide is a diuretic that would not be helpful for someone with urinary incontinence unless absolutely necessary for some other health condition. Finasteride and Doxazosin are both drugs that are prescribed for prostate enlargement and not appropriate for this particular scenario.

24. D: Aseptic technique is the recommended technique to use when inserting a urinary catheter and will help in the prevention of catheter-associated urinary tract infections (CAUTIs). Sanitary and clean techniques are lower on the scale of techniques and therefore not adequate. Sterile technique is usually used in surgical procedures in which an environment without micro-organisms present is desirable.

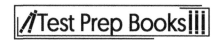

25. A: The patient with tented T waves, widening QRS complex, and deep S waves is likely experiencing hyperkalemia. Any potassium that is being infused should be stopped, the doctor notified, and correction of the imbalance performed immediately. Hyper- and hyponatremia are not applicable here, though they are both examples of electrolyte imbalances. Hypokalemia presents differently, with weakness, polyuria, hyperexcitable cardiac cells, and muscle cramping.

26. B: The nurse suspects that the IV has infiltrated, meaning the catheter tip has become dislodged and IV medication and/or fluids are leaking into the surrounding tissues. The nurse should stop the infusion, remove the IV, and dress the site. An allergic reaction or infection would be warm, not cold, due to the inflammatory response present in such conditions. This is not a normal assessment of a peripheral IV.

27. C: Removing the pillows from the bed is not the best option, as these are used to support the patient's limbs and reduce pressure to bony prominences. All the other interventions, including encouraging early mobility, proper nutrition, and turning and repositioning the patient every two hours will help prevent the development of pressure ulcers.

28. D: An infected wound will become reddened, inflamed, and discharge pus. A surgical wound should be clean with approximated boundaries. A trauma wound may be irregularly shaped and large. A healing wound develops scabbing, and possibly scar tissue, but should not appear as the wound described.

29. D: Unless facility policy describes otherwise, nurses are not to re-suture incisions. The surgeon or first-assist usually takes charge of such duties, as they are specially trained to do so. The critical care nurse will monitor the wound, assessing for signs of infection, maintain a clean dressing daily or as prescribed, and apply prescribed medications.

30. B: The highest priority in this patient is stopping the flow of blood out of her body. Nothing else can be addressed until this is performed. Fluid resuscitation is highly important, but useless if the bleeding continues. Monitoring for infection will happen later. Assessing for organ damage is ongoing, but ultimately secondary to stopping active bleeding.

Musculoskeletal/Neurology/Psychosocial

Musculoskeletal

Infections

Infectious arthritis may be acute or chronic. In acute cases, the infection can spread in three ways: the bloodstream can carry an infection from another part of the body to the bones; direct invasion can occur through open fractures, surgery, or objects that pierce the bone; and infections can be transferred from soft tissues near the bone, or via artificial joint.

In young adults and adolescents, *Neisseria gonorrhoeae* is the most common cause of acute infectious arthritis, and results when *N. gonorrhoeae* spreads from infected mucosal surfaces (cervix, urethra, rectum, pharynx) via the bloodstream. In adults, most acute joint infections result from bacteria and are classified as gonococcal or nongonococcal. This distinction is important because gonococcal infections are far less destructive to the joint. In adults overall, Staphylococcus aureus tends to be the most frequent cause of infectious arthritis and MRSA has become the primary culprit.

A chronic case of infectious arthritis usually involves mycobacteria, bacteria, or fungal organisms and often occurs in patients on immunosuppressive therapy. Patients with Lyme Disease caused by borrelia burgdorferi may present only with acute monarthritis or oligoarthritis, which may recur if left untreated. Cultures of synovial fluid surrounding the joint are taken to confirm or rule out the causative organism, and determine if infectious arthritis is occurring. The treatment plan for a patient may include antibiotic or antifungal drug therapy, as well as possible drainage of the joint.

Infections are more common in prosthetic joints than in natural joints. They are frequently caused by perioperative inoculations of bacteria into the joint or by postoperative bacteremia resulting from skin infection, pneumonia, dental procedures, invasive instrumentation, UTI, or possibly falls. The diagnosis of infection in a prosthetic joint often requires a combination of clinical, microbiologic, pathologic, and imaging criteria. Communication between a sinus tract and the prosthesis may also be considered diagnostic of infection. Synovial fluid should be sampled for cell count and culture. X-rays may show loosening of the prosthesis or periosteal reaction but are not diagnostic. Technetium-99m bone scanning and indium-labeled WBC scanning are more sensitive than plain x-rays but may lack specificity in the immediate postoperative period. Ultimately, periprosthetic tissue collected at the time of surgery may be sent for culture and histologic analysis.

Treatment of prosthetic joint infection is prolonged and usually involves arthrotomy for prosthesis removal and debridement of all cement, abscesses, and devitalized tissues. Debridement is followed by immediate prosthesis revision or placement of an antibiotic-impregnated spacer and then delayed implantation of a new prosthesis using antibiotic-impregnated cement. Infection develops in 38% of replacement prostheses, whether replaced immediately or after delay. Joint infections develop within one year of surgery in two-thirds of cases. Osteomyelitis may occur where a piece of metal has been surgically attached to a bone. The organisms may be carried into the area of bone surrounding the artificial joint during the operation to replace the joint, or the infection may occur later.

Osteomyelitis is a destructive infection of the bone, often caused by Staphylococcus aureus. A patient presenting with bone pain, fever, and malaise should be diagnosed using a CT scan or MRI. Broad spectrum antibiotic therapy is prescribed, based on the results of bone tissue cultures. Osteomyelitis occurs most commonly in young children and in older people, but all age groups are at risk.

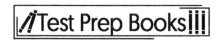

Osteomyelitis is also more likely to occur in people with serious medical conditions. When a bone becomes infected, the bone marrow swells. As the swollen tissue presses against the rigid outer wall of the bone, the blood vessels in the bone marrow are compressed, which restricts blood supply to the bone.

Most osteomyelitis results from direct invasion or infections in nearby soft tissue such as deep pressure sores. Osteomyelitis may also result from an infection in nearby soft tissue. The infection spreads to the bone after several days or weeks. When osteomyelitis results from infections in nearby soft tissues or direct invasion by an organism, the area over the bone swells and becomes painful. Abscesses may form in the surrounding tissue. Such an infection may start in an area damaged by an injury or surgery, radiation therapy, or cancer or in a skin ulcer (particularly a foot ulcer) caused by poor circulation or diabetes. A sinus, gum, or tooth infection may spread to the skull.

Infections of the vertebrae are referred to as vertebral osteomyelitis. People who are older, are debilitated, have sickle cell disease, undergo kidney dialysis, or inject drugs using nonsterile needles are particularly susceptible to vertebral osteomyelitis. Vertebral osteomyelitis usually develops gradually, causing persistent back pain and tenderness when touched. Pain worsens with movement and is not relieved by resting, applying heat, or taking analgesics. Fever, usually the most obvious sign of an infection, is often absent.

Chronic osteomyelitis may develop if osteomyelitis is not treated successfully. It is a persistent infection, undetectable for a long time, causing no symptoms for months or years. Chronic osteomyelitis causes bone pain, recurring infections in the soft tissue over the bone, and constant or intermittent drainage of pus through the skin. Such drainage occurs when a sinus tract forms from the infected bone to the skin surface and pus drains through the sinus tract.

Symptoms during a physical examination may suggest osteomyelitis and diagnosis is confirmed through CT, MRI or bone scan as well as erythrocyte sedimentation rate (ESR) and level of C-reactive protein.

Functional Issues

Walking without assistance requires attention, muscle strength and effective motor control to coordinate the sensory input and muscle contractions. Some elements of gait normally change with aging while others do not. Gait velocity remains stable until about age 70, then declines about 15% per decade for usual gait and 20% per decade for fast walking. Gait velocity slows because elderly people take shorter steps at the same cadence. The most likely reason for shortened step length is weakness of the calf muscles, which propel the body forward. Calf muscle strength is substantially decreased in elderly people; however, they compensate for decreased lower calf power by using their hip flexor and extensor muscles more than young adults.

Elderly people walk with greater downward pelvic rotation and increased lumbar lordosis. This posture change is usually due to a combination of weak abdominal muscles, tight hip flexor muscles, and increased abdominal fat. Elderly people also walk with toes out about 5°, generally due to a loss of hip internal rotation or in order to increase lateral stability. A number of disorders can contribute to dysfunctional or unsafe gait, including neurologic and musculoskeletal disorders, dementias, movement and cerebellar disorders, and sensory or motor neuropathies.

Difficulty initiating or maintaining gait may occur. When patients first start walking, their feet may appear stuck to the floor, typically because patients do not shift their weight to one foot to allow the other foot to move forward. This problem may represent isolated gait initiation failure, Parkinson disease, or frontal or subcortical disease. Festination, which occurs with Parkinson disease, is a progressive quickening of steps where patients may break into a run to prevent falling forward. Once gait is initiated, steps should be continuous, with little variability in the timing of the steps. Freezing, stopping, or almost stopping usually suggests a cautious gait, a fear of falling, or a frontal lobe gait disorder. Scuffing the feet is not normal and is a risk factor for tripping.

Foot drop causes toe dragging or a stepping gait. It may be secondary to anterior tibialis weakness, spasticity of calf muscles, or lowering of the pelvis due to muscle weakness of the proximal muscles on the stance side. Arm swing may be reduced or absent in Parkinson disease and vascular dementias. Arm swing disorders may also be adverse effects of dopamine-blocking drugs. Assistive devices provide stability but also affect gait. Use of walkers often results in a flexed posture and discontinuous gait, particularly if the walker has no wheels.

In addition to the standard medical history, elderly patients should be asked about gait-related issues. Routine gait assessment can be done by a primary care practitioner and physical therapy professionals may be called in to perform a mobility assessment. A CT or MRI of the brain is often done, particularly when there is poor gait initiation, chaotic cadence, or the appearance of a very stiff gait. These tests help identify lacunar infarcts, white matter disease, and focal atrophy

Deconditioning is a complex process of physiological change following a period of inactivity, bedrest or sedentary lifestyle. It results in functional losses in such areas as mental status, degree of continence and ability to accomplish activities of daily living. Clinical studies have shown that the bedbound patient suffers a 20% decrease in muscle strength per week and a 50% decrease in muscle strength after a month in bed. There is also a 3% loss of muscle mass within the thigh muscles within 7 days. Within 7 days the muscle fibers & connective tissues are maintained in a shortened position and contractures begin within 3 weeks.

Elderly patients, patients with cognitive dysfunction, and patients whose illnesses have left them debilitated and weak, are at a considerable risk of falling. Falls are a leading cause of injury and accidental deaths in the elderly. Gait and balance disorders, functional impairments, visual defects, cognitive impairments, and use of psychotropic medications are the most important risk factors for falls. Primary prevention of falls includes high levels of physical activity, even in patients with disease. Secondary prevention includes improving gait along with resistance and balance training. The effects of an active lifestyle on mood and confidence are probably as important as their effect on physiology.

All critical care patients should be considered fall risks. Environmental factors such as the lighting of the room, objects on the floor, and proximity to the call light must all be factored in to help prevent a fall. Most hospitals have a fall risk policy and a method to identify the high risk patients. Indicators such as yellow fall arm bands, signs on doors, or yellow slippers can all alert the staff that the patient is a fall risk. The critical care nurse should work closely with the family and caregivers so that patients at risk can have the monitoring they need to prevent a fall. Bed alarms and sitters may be indicated.

Neurology

Brain Death
When the functioning capacity of the brain is lost but the heart and the lungs continue artificially, this is called brain death. The cerebrum and brain stem no longer signal spontaneous respiration and there are no brain stem reflexes. The concept of brain death developed because ventilators and drugs can continue cardiopulmonary and other body functions despite complete cessation of all cerebral activity.

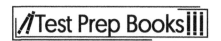

The concept that the brain determines a person's death has been accepted legally and culturally in most of the world. The following, which is the American Academy of Neurology's Guidelines for Brain Death Determination, is the pathway most hospitals use for their policy:

1. Establish proximate cause and irreversibility of coma and monitor the patient for an appropriate waiting period in order to exclude the possibility of recovery.

2. Initiate the hospital policy for notifying the patient's Surrogate Decision-maker.

3. Conduct and document the clinical assessment of brain stem reflexes.

4. Perform and document the apnea test. An apnea test of a minimum of 8 min shows no respiratory movements with a documented increase in Paco2 of > 20 mm Hg from pretest baseline. Apnea testing is done by disconnecting the ventilator from the endotracheal tube. Oxygen (6 L/min) can be supplied by diffusion from a cannula placed through the endotracheal tube. Despite the ventilatory stimulus of the passively rising Paco2, no spontaneous respirations are seen over an 8- to 12-min period.

5. Perform ancillary testing, if indicated. Sometimes EEG, brain vascular imaging, or both.

6. If the individual's religious or moral objection to the brain death standard is known, implement hospital policies for reasonable accommodation.

7. Certify brain death.

8. Discontinue cardio-respiratory support in accordance with hospital policies, including those for organ donation. Brain death is loss of function of the entire cerebrum and brain stem, resulting in coma, no spontaneous respiration, and loss of all brain stem reflexes. Spinal reflexes, including deep tendon, plantar flexion, and withdrawal reflexes, may remain. Recovery does not occur.

After brain death is confirmed, all supporting cardiac and respiratory treatments are ended. Terminal arrhythmias result and spinal motor reflexes may occur during terminal apnea; they include arching of the back, neck turning, stiffening of the legs, and upper extremity flexion. Family members who wish to be present when the ventilator is shut off need to be warned of such reflex movements. A patient diagnosed as brain dead is removed from all cardiopulmonary support and palliation is given until the patient expires.

Encephalopathy

Encephalopathy is a general term that means brain disease, damage, or malfunction, with the major symptom being an altered mental state. Encephalopathy is often considered a complication of a primary problem. In most cases, the word encephalopathy is preceded by a term that describes the reason, cause, or special conditions of the patient that leads to brain malfunction. For example, anoxic encephalopathy means brain damage due to lack of oxygen, and hepatic encephalopathy means brain malfunction due to liver disease.

A broad spectrum of symptoms occur that can range from mild (some memory loss or subtle personality changes) to severe (dementia, seizures, coma, or death). In general, encephalopathy shows itself as an altered mental state sometimes accompanied by physical manifestations.

Chronic traumatic encephalopathy (CTE) describes a gradual degeneration in brain function due to repeated head injuries that causes both symptomatic and asymptomatic concussions. Once the initial symptoms of concussion have faded, months and years later, new symptoms occur. CTE symptoms start slowly and creep up on the patient. Initially, there may be concentration and memory problems with episodes of disorientation and confusion, dizziness, and headache. It is as if the concussion symptoms were starting to return even without a new head injury. This type of encephalopathy is usually irreversible. CTE is common in athletes such as boxers and football players who have received several blows to the head during their career. Symptom management and improving quality of life for the patient and the caregivers is the priority.

Although numerous causes of encephalopathy are known, the majority of cases arise from several major categories: infection (HIV, Neisseria meningitides, herpes, and hepatitis B and hepatitis C), liver damage (alcohol and toxins), brain anoxia, or brain cell destruction (including trauma), and kidney failure (uremic).

Hemorrhage

Intracranial Hemorrhage (ICH)

Although most intracerebral hemorrhages (ICH) occur in the basal ganglia, cerebral lobes, cerebellum, or pons, they can also occur in other parts of the brain stem or in the midbrain. ICH usually presents as rupture of a small arteriosclerotic artery that has been weakened by chronic arterial hypertension. Such hemorrhages are usually large and catastrophic. Risk factors that contribute to arteriosclerotic hypertensive intracerebral hemorrhages include smoking, obesity, and a diet high in saturated fats, trans fats, and calories. Use of cocaine or, other sympathomimetic drugs can cause transient severe hypertension leading to hemorrhage. ICH occurs less frequently from these causes: congenital aneurysm, arteriovenous or other vascular malformation, trauma, mycotic aneurysm, brain infarct, brain tumor, excessive anticoagulation, blood dyscrasia, intracranial arterial dissection, or a vasculitic disorder.

Symptoms typically begin with sudden headache during activity. However, headache may be mild or absent in the elderly. Loss of consciousness is common, often within seconds or a few minutes. Nausea, vomiting, delirium, and focal or generalized seizures are also common. Neurologic deficits are usually sudden and progressive. Large hemorrhages, when located in the hemispheres, cause hemiparesis; when located in the posterior fossa, they cause cerebellar or brain stem deficits (eye deviation, pinpoint pupils, coma). Large hemorrhages are fatal within a few days in about half of patients.

Arteriovenous malformations (AVMs) are tangled, dilated blood vessels in which arteries flow directly into veins. AVMs occur most often at the junction of cerebral arteries, usually within the parenchyma of the frontal-parietal region, frontal lobe, lateral cerebellum, or overlying occipital lobe. AVMs also can occur within the dura. An AVM can bleed or directly compress brain tissue, resulting in seizures or ischemia. Neuroimaging may detect them incidentally; contrast or non-contrast CT can usually detect AVMs > 1 cm, but the diagnosis is confirmed with MRI. Occasionally, a cranial bruit suggests an AVM. Conventional angiography is required for definitive diagnosis and determination of whether the lesion is operable. Superficial AVMs > 3 cm in diameter are usually removed with microsurgery, radiosurgery, and endovascular surgery. AVMs that are deep or < 3 cm in diameter are treated with stereotactic radiosurgery, endovascular therapy or coagulation with focused proton beams.

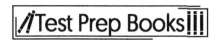

Intraventricular Hemorrhage (IVH)

Intraventricular hemorrhage (IVH) is a bleeding into the brain's ventricular system, where the cerebrospinal fluid is produced and circulates through towards the subarachnoid space. It can result from physical trauma or from a stroke. IVH are graded as follows: Grade I, bleeding confined to periventricular area; Grade II, intraventricular bleeding 10-50% of ventricular area on sagittal view; Grade III, intraventricular bleeding with >50% of ventricular area; Grade IV, directly involves brain tissue and includes hydrocephalus

In adults, an intraventricular hemorrhage usually occurs along with a cerebral hemorrhage. Premature babies have immature or poorly developed brain tissue, which predisposes them to have spontaneous intraventricular hemorrhage. Early respiratory distress syndrome and cerebral palsy are associated with this type of bleed in neonates.

Symptoms of intraventricular hemorrhage in adults are similar to those of intracranial bleeds, with headache, neurological deficits, and nausea and vomiting being most prevalent. Diagnosis and treatment also include CT scanning, hemodynamic monitoring and stabilization and potential surgical intervention to drain hemorrhaging blood that is compressing brain tissue.

Subarachnoid

Emergency management of subarachnoid hemorrhage (SAH) is critical; an estimated 10-15% of patients die before reaching the hospital. Mortality rate reaches as high as 40% within the first week, and about 50% die in the first 6 months. Subarachnoid hemorrhage is bleeding between the arachnoid and pia mater, generally caused by head trauma. Less common causes are aneurysms, arteriovenous malformations, and bleeding disorders. A patient experiencing a subarachnoid hemorrhage presents with headache, orbital pain, dizziness, double vision or diplopia, and/or loss of vision. Some patients may experience prodromal symptoms such as sensory or motor disturbances, seizures, ptosis, bruits, and/or dysphasia. The nurse may find the patient tachycardic, feverish, hypertensive, with swelling around the eyes and hemorrhage of the retinas.

Spontaneous (primary) subarachnoid hemorrhage usually results from ruptured aneurysms. A congenital intracranial saccular or berry aneurysm is the cause in about 85% of patients. Bleeding may stop spontaneously. Aneurysmal hemorrhage may occur at any age but is most common from age 40 to 65.

Aneurysms are focal dilations in arteries that occur in about 5% of people. Common contributing factors include arteriosclerosis, hypertension, and hereditary connective tissue disorders. Brain aneurysms are most often < 2.5 cm in diameter and noncircumferential. Most aneurysms occur along the middle or anterior cerebral arteries or the communicating branches of the circle of Willis, particularly at arterial bifurcations. Most aneurysms are asymptomatic, but a few cause symptoms by compressing adjacent structures. Ocular palsies, diplopia, squint, or orbital pain may indicate pressure on the 3rd, 4th, 5th, or 6th cranial nerves.

Aneurysms may bleed into the subarachnoid space, causing subarachnoid hemorrhage. Before rupture, aneurysms occasionally cause sentinel headaches due to painful expansion of the aneurysm or to blood leaking into the subarachnoid space. Actual rupture causes a sudden severe headache called a thunderclap headache. CT is performed to image the brain tissue and blood pressure will need to be stabilized with IV beta blockers, followed by a visit to the surgical suite to clip the ruptured aneurysm. The patient who has had a subarachnoid bleed must be monitored for the development of complications such as re-bleed, vasospasm, seizures, hyponatremia, and hydrocephalus.

Ischemic Stroke

Ischemic stroke is sudden neurologic deficits that result from focal cerebral ischemia associated with permanent brain infarction. Common causes are (from most to least common) atherothrombotic occlusion of large arteries; cerebral embolism; non-thrombotic occlusion of small, deep cerebral arteries (lacunar infarction); and proximal arterial stenosis with hypotension that decreases cerebral blood flow in arterial watershed zones (hemodynamic stroke). Diagnosis is clinical, but CT or MRI is done to exclude hemorrhage and confirm the presence and extent of stroke. Thrombolytic therapy may be useful acutely in certain patients. Depending on the cause of stroke, carotid endarterectomy or stenting, antiplatelet drugs, or warfarin may help reduce risk of subsequent strokes.

Ischemia usually results from atherothrombotic occlusion of large arteries. Atheromas, particularly if ulcerated, predispose to thrombi, can occur in any major cerebral artery and are common at areas of turbulent flow, particularly at the carotid bifurcation. Less common causes of thrombosis include vascular inflammation secondary to disorders such as acute or chronic meningitis, vasculitic disorders, and syphilis; dissection of intracranial arteries or the aorta; hypercoagulability disorders; polycythemia, thrombocytosis, hemoglobinopathies, and plasma cell disorders; and rare disorders (e.g., fibromuscular dysplasia, moyamoya disease, Binswanger disease). Older oral contraceptive formulations increase risk of thrombosis. In children, sickle cell disease is a common cause of ischemic stroke.

Inadequate blood flow in a single brain artery can often be compensated for by an efficient collateral system, particularly between the carotid and vertebral arteries via anastomoses at the circle of Willis and, to a lesser extent, between major arteries supplying the cerebral hemispheres. However, normal variations in the circle of Willis and in the caliber of various collateral vessels, atherosclerosis, and other acquired arterial lesions can interfere with collateral flow, increasing the chance that blockage of one artery will cause brain ischemia.

Embolic strokes often occur during the day; headache may precede neurologic deficits. Thrombi tend to occur during the night and thus are first noticed on awakening. Deterioration during the first 48 to 72 hours after onset of symptoms, particularly progressively impaired consciousness, results more often from cerebral edema than from extension of the infarct. Unless the infarct is large or extensive, function commonly improves within the first few days; further improvement occurs gradually for up to 1 year.

Diagnosis of ischemic stroke is suggested by sudden neurologic deficits referable to a specific arterial territory. For vascular causes, testing may include magnetic resonance angiography (MRA), CT angiography (CTA), carotid and transcranial duplex ultrasonography, and conventional angiography. The scale of the stroke is measured using the National Institutes of Health Stroke Scale (NIHSS). If an ischemic stroke is suspected, CT scanning will be ordered to visualize the area of ischemia and determine if there are any blockages of blood vessels. A patient who has had an ischemic stroke will be put on platelet anti-aggregants, anti-hypertensives, and statins, and will receive lifestyle recommendations to prevent future strokes.

For thrombotic disorders blood testing typically includes CBC, platelet count, PT/PTT, fasting blood glucose, and lipid profile. Depending on which causes are clinically suspected, additional tests may include measurement of homocysteine; testing for thrombotic disorders (antiphospholipid antibodies, protein S, protein C, antithrombin III, factor V Leidenantinuclear antibodies); rheumatoid factor, ESR, syphilis serologic testing, Hb electrophoresis, and a urine drug screen for cocaine and amphetamines. Stroke severity and progression are often assessed using standardized measures such as the NIHSS. Thrombolytic therapy may be useful acutely in certain patients and depending on the cause of stroke,

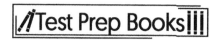

carotid endarterectomy, stenting, antiplatelet drugs, or warfarin may help reduce risk of subsequent strokes.

The following behaviors are considered modifiable risk factors associated with increased risk of ischemic stroke: smoking, abdominal obesity, alcoholism, lack of physical activity, and cocaine and amphetamine use. Predisposing medical factors include: diabetes, insulin resistance, hypertension, dyslipidemia, depression, heart disorders, hypercoagulability, and vasculitis. Prior stroke, older age, and family history of stroke are considered non-modifiable factors.

Ischemia usually results from thrombi or emboli. A patient experiencing a stroke will display the following signs and symptoms: hemi-, mono-, or quadri-paresis, in which they are partially or fully paralyzed; hemisensory deficits; visual loss in one or both eyes; double vision; facial droop; nystagmus; aphasia; and decrease in level of consciousness. All symptoms of stroke are reflective of the part of the brain tissue that has been affected by ischemic conditions.

There are certain conditions that may mimic an ischemic attack, such as a TIA, in which the blockage of blood flow only occurs for a short time before perfusion is restored, and no lasting damage occurs. It is important to establish that an ischemic stroke is in fact the true diagnosis before treatment options can be carefully selected. If it is a true ischemic stroke, re-perfusion therapies will be chosen, in which fibrinolytic agents will be administered to try and destroy the clot causing the ischemia. These fibrinolytic agents are potent and could cause severe bleeding and internal hemorrhage if not administered and monitored with great care.

Neurologic Infectious Diseases

Encephalitis, an inflammation of the parenchyma of the brain, should be suspected in patients with unexplained alterations in mental status. Acute disseminated encephalomyelitis is brain and spinal cord inflammation caused by a hypersensitivity reaction a foreign protein. Both disorders are usually triggered by viruses and are classified as follows: Epidemic (arbovirus, echovirus, coxsackievirus); sporadic (cytomegalovirus, herpes simplex, varicella-zoster, rabies, or mumps virus); or mosquito-borne (West Nile, St. Louis, Eastern and Western equine, Zika).

Symptoms include fever, headache, and altered mental status, often accompanied by seizures and focal neurologic deficits. A GI or respiratory prodrome may precede these symptoms. Meningeal signs are typically mild and less prominent than other manifestations. Status epilepticus, particularly convulsive status epilepticus, or coma suggests severe brain inflammation and a poor prognosis. Olfactory seizures, manifested as an aura of foul smells (rotten eggs, burnt meat), indicate temporal lobe involvement and suggest HSV encephalitis.

Diagnosis requires CSF analysis and neuroimaging. Treatment is supportive and may include antiviral drugs. Clinical presentation and differential diagnoses may suggest certain diagnostic tests, but MRI and CSF analysis (including PCR for HSV and other viruses) are usually done, typically with other, serologic tests to identify the causative virus. Despite extensive testing, the cause of many cases of encephalitis remains unknown.

Recovery from viral encephalitis may take a long time. Mortality rate varies with cause, but severity of epidemics due to the same virus varies during different years. Permanent neurologic deficits are common among patients who survive severe infection.

Meningitis is inflammation of the meninges and subarachnoid space that may result from infections, other medical disorders, or reactions to drugs. Meningitis may be classified as acute, subacute, chronic, or recurrent and by its cause; bacteria, viruses, fungi, and protozoa. The most clinically useful categories of meningitis will be used here: acute bacterial, viral, noninfectious, recurrent, subacute, and chronic.

Acute bacterial meningitis is serious and rapidly progressive. Aseptic meningitis is an older term used synonymously with viral meningitis; however, it usually refers to acute meningitis caused by anything other than meningococcus or streptococcus. Viral and noninfectious infections are usually self-limited. Subacute and chronic meningitis usually follows a slower course and makes diagnosis difficult. Symptoms vary in severity and acuity; however, all types of meningitis present with headache, fever, nuchal rigidity, and lethargy. Nuchal rigidity can be distinguished from neck stiffness because the neck can usually be rotated but cannot be flexed.

Neurosurgery

Neurosurgery, the practice of surgery on the neurological system and its structures, may be performed for numerous different diagnoses. Procedures can be performed via stereotactic techniques, conventional open surgery, and microsurgery. Microscopic surgeries can include laminectomy, microdiscectomy, and artificial disc replacement. There are hundreds of different types of neurosurgery procedures ranging from the minor to complicated. The critical care nurse might see patients recovering from the following surgeries.

- Anterior Cervical Discectomy and Fusion: Because it is not generally safe to access herniated discs in the neck from the back, treatment of these usually requires this anterior approach.

- Craniotomy: Surgical treatment of some brain diseases or tumor removal.

- Epilepsy Surgery: When a patient does not respond adequately to medications, there are different types of procedures that are used to diagnose and treat epilepsy.

- Laminectomy: A procedure to access and decompress the spine

- Lumbar Puncture: The gold standard test for diagnosing meningitis, a lumbar puncture may be used in the diagnosis of a number of different diseases of the nervous system.

- Microdiscectomy: One of the most common procedures used to treat a disease of the nervous system, this procedure is the way that most herniated discs in the lumbar spine are treated.

- Pituitary Tumor Surgery: Most pituitary adenomas, benign tumors of the pituitary gland, are treated by surgery through a route called the transsphenoidal approach.

- Spinal Fusion: Fusion of the spine may be necessary in a number of spinal disease conditions, from degenerative disease to trauma.

- Ventriculoperitoneal Shunt: One of the classic treatments for hydrocephalus, a shunt is an internal implant that helps divert fluid from the brain.

- Ventriculostomy: A tube placed into the fluid spaces within the brain, is a common procedure that may be used in a number of different clinical situations

Seizure Disorders

A seizure is an abnormal, unregulated electrical discharge that occurs within the brain's cortical gray matter and interrupts normal brain function. A seizure typically causes altered awareness, abnormal

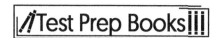

sensations, and convulsions. Diagnosis may be clinical and involves results of neuroimaging, laboratory testing, and EEG for new-onset seizures or anticonvulsant levels for previously diagnosed seizure disorders. Treatment includes elimination of the cause if possible, anticonvulsants, and surgery.

Epilepsy (also called epileptic seizure disorder) is a chronic brain disorder characterized by recurrent ($\geq$ 2) seizures that are unprovoked and that occur > 24 h apart. A single seizure is not considered an epileptic seizure. Epilepsy is often idiopathic, but various brain disorders, such as malformations, strokes, and tumors, can cause symptomatic epilepsy. Symptomatic epilepsy is epilepsy due to a known cause (brain tumor, stroke). The seizures it causes are called symptomatic epileptic seizures and are most common among neonates and the elderly.

Nonepileptic seizures are provoked by a temporary disorder or stressor, such as metabolic disorders, CNS infections, cardiovascular disorders, drug toxicity or withdrawal, or psychogenic disorders. By age of onset, the common causes of seizures are: before age 2, fever, birth or developmental defects, birth injuries, and metabolic disorders; ages 2 to 14, idiopathic seizure disorders; adults, cerebral trauma, alcohol withdrawal, tumors, strokes, and an unknown cause in 50%; the elderly, tumors and strokes.

Seizures are classified as generalized or partial. In generalized seizures, the aberrant electrical discharge diffusely involves the entire cortex of both hemispheres from the onset, and consciousness is usually lost. Generalized seizures result most often from metabolic disorders and sometimes from genetic disorders. In partial seizures, the excess neuronal discharge occurs in one cerebral cortex, and most often results from structural abnormalities. Partial (focal) seizures may evolve into a generalized seizure (called secondary generalization), which causes loss of consciousness. Secondary generalization occurs when a partial seizure spreads and activates the entire cerebrum bilaterally. Activation may occur so rapidly that the initial partial seizure is not clinically apparent or is very brief.

Auras are simple partial seizures that begin focally. Auras may consist of motor activity or sensory, autonomic, or psychic sensations. Most seizures end spontaneously in 1 to 2 min. A postictal state often follows generalized seizures; it is characterized by deep sleep, headache, confusion, and muscle soreness; this state lasts from minutes to hours. Sometimes the postictal state includes **Todd paralysis**, a transient neurologic deficit, usually weakness, of the limb contralateral to the seizure focus. Most patients appear neurologically normal between seizures, although high doses of the drugs used to treat seizure disorders, particularly anticonvulsants, can reduce alertness. Any progressive mental deterioration is usually related to the neurologic disorder that caused the seizures rather than to the seizures themselves.

Testing is done routinely, but normal results do not necessarily exclude a seizure disorder. Thus, the diagnosis may ultimately be clinical. Testing depends on results of the history and neurologic examination. If patients have a known seizure disorder and examination results are normal or unchanged, little testing is required except blood anticonvulsant levels. Additional testing is indicated if patients have symptoms or signs of a treatable disorder such as trauma, infection, or a metabolic disorder. If seizures are new-onset or if examination results are abnormal for the first time, neuroimaging is required. Patients with new-onset seizures or atypical manifestations also require laboratory testing, including blood tests (serum electrolytes, BUN, creatinine, glucose, Ca, Mg, and K levels), and liver function tests. Other tests may be done based on disorders that are suspected clinically.

Unreported use of recreational drugs that can cause or contribute to seizures: Drug screens may be done, although this practice is controversial because positive results do not indicate causality and test results can be inaccurate.

Follow-up MRI is recommended when CT is negative. It provides better resolution of brain tumors and abscesses and can detect cortical dysplasias, cerebral venous thrombosis, and herpes encephalitis. MRI can detect some common causes of seizures, such as malformations of cortical development in young children and mesial temporal sclerosis, traumatic gliosis, and small tumors in adults.

EEG is critical in the diagnosis of epileptic seizures, particularly of complex partial or absence status epilepticus, when EEG may be the most definitive indication of a seizure. EEG may detect epileptiform abnormalities (spikes, sharp waves, spike and slow-wave complexes, polyspike and slow-wave complexes). Epileptiform abnormalities may be bilateral, symmetric, and synchronous in patients with primarily generalized seizures and may be localized in patients with partial seizures. EEG findings may include the following:

With treatment, seizures are eliminated in one third of patients with epileptic seizures, and frequency of seizures is reduced by > 50% in another third. About 60% of patients whose seizures are well-controlled by drugs can eventually stop the drugs and remain seizure-free. Epileptic seizures are considered resolved when patients have been seizure-free for 10 years and have not taken anticonvulsants for the last five years of that time period.

If the cause cannot be corrected or identified, anticonvulsants are often required, particularly after a second seizure; usefulness of anticonvulsants after a single seizure is controversial, and risks and benefits should be discussed with the patient. Because the risk of a subsequent seizure is low, drugs may be withheld until a second seizure occurs, particularly in children. In children, certain anticonvulsants cause important behavior and learning problems.

Most seizures remit spontaneously in several minutes or less and do not require emergency drug treatment. However, status epilepticus and most seizures lasting > 5 min require drugs to terminate the seizures, with monitoring of respiratory status. Endotracheal intubation is necessary if there is any indication of airway compromise. The sooner anticonvulsant therapy is started, the better and the more easily seizures are controlled. IV access should be quickly obtained, and patients are given lorazepam 0.05 to 0.1 mg/kg IV (typically a 4-mg IV dose for adults) at a rate of 2 mg/min. Larger doses are sometimes required. After lorazepam is given, a second, longer-acting anticonvulsant is indicated.

There is no consensus or evidence-based guideline indicating which longer-acting anticonvulsant is preferred. Many experts choose one of the following: Fosphenytoin 15 to 20 PE (phenytoin equivalents)/kg IV, given at a rate of 100 to 150 PE/min

Anticonvulsants may be required indefinitely, but many types of seizures (most febrile seizures, seizures due to alcohol withdrawal, seizures that do not recur) do not require treatment with anticonvulsants. No single drug controls all types of seizures and some patients require multiple drugs. The drugs preferred vary according to type of seizure

About 10 to 20% of patients have intractable seizures refractory to medical treatment and are potential surgical candidates. If seizures originate from a focal, resectable area in the brain, resection of the epileptic focus usually improves seizure control markedly. If the focus is in the anteromesial temporal lobe, resection eliminates seizures in about 60% of patients. After surgical resection, some patients remain seizure-free without taking anticonvulsants, but many still require the drugs, but in reduced

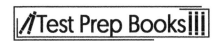

doses and possibly as monotherapy. Because surgery requires extensive testing and monitoring, these patients are best treated in specialized epilepsy centers.

Space-Occupying Lesions/Brain Tumors

Space occupying lesions (SOLs) of the central nervous system can pursue a serious clinical course even when they are inflammatory or benign. SOL are growths within the skull, which present with common symptoms and signs. The most common causes are metastatic brain tumors. The primary brain tumors are astrocytoma, glioblastoma, olygodendroglyoma, and ependuymoma, which all have less than a five-year survival rate. Meningeoma is a benign tumor which is twice as common in women. Brain aneurisms, abscesses, and subdural hematomas are all benign.

The presenting symptoms of SOL are those of increased intracranial pressure: focal neurological signs, seizures, headache, nausea and vomiting, behavioral changes, paralysis, and visual disturbances. Loss of vision and combinations of symptoms can also occur, depending upon the brain region involved in the process. Localizing syndromes differentiate lesions in the occipital, temporal, frontal, and parietal regions.

Radiology is the primary assessment method prior to a surgical diagnosis. Radiological techniques allow precise localization for a stereotactic biopsy. When there is a radiologic impression of an SOL, histological confirmation is required.

The treatment of the brain tumor is based on severity of the tumor. Mannitol is helpful in treating brain herniation and Dexamethasone may be prescribed to decrease the intracranial pressure. Depending on the location of the tumor and intensity of the disease, excision may be necessary. Radiation therapy and/or chemotherapy and stereotactic radiosurgery are also treatment options.

Traumatic Brain Injuries

Traumatic brain injury, often referred to as TBI, is often an acute event. Because the brain defines the identity, the consequences of a brain injury can affect all aspects of the patient's life, especially the personality. A brain does not heal like other injuries. There is a popular quote that says *recovery from a brain injury lasts a lifetime*, and it's also possible that you never fully recover. No two brain injuries are alike and the consequence of two similar injuries may be very different. Symptoms may appear right away or may not be present for days or weeks after the injury. In these cases, as well as others, the patient with brain trauma does not realize that a brain injury has occurred. The TBI may either temporarily or permanently cause damage, depending on the severity of the blow to the head. TBIs occur during motor vehicle crashes, falls, or blows to the head, among many other potential causes.

An open TBI is one in which the scalp and skull are penetrated and the tissue beneath is exposed. A closed TBI occurs from violent shaking or blows to the head, but the skull is not penetrated. During both types of TBI, blood vessels can tear and leak and hematomas may form.

A TBI is also classified as either mild or severe. A brain injury can be classified as mild if loss of consciousness and/or confusion and disorientation is shorter than 30 minutes. While MRI and CAT scans are often normal, the individual has cognitive problems such as headache, difficulty thinking, memory problems, attention deficits, mood swings, and frustration. These injuries are commonly overlooked. Even though this type of TBI is called mild, the effect on the patient and family can be devastating.

Severe brain injury is associated with loss of consciousness for more than 30 minutes and memory loss longer than 24 hours. The deficits range from impairment of higher level cognitive functions to comatose states. Survivors may have limited function of arms or legs, abnormal speech or language, loss of thinking ability or emotional problems. The range of injuries and degree of recovery varies with each individual

The effects of a TBI can be profound. Individuals with severe injuries can be left in long-term unresponsive states. For many people with a severe TBI, long-term rehabilitation is often necessary to maximize function and independence. Even with a mild TBI, changes in brain function can have a dramatic impact on memory, family, job, social and community interaction. Treatment depends upon the stage at which the TBI is discovered. Acute care, surgery, rehabilitation and supportive care are all options that are dependent upon the stage of recovery.

Concussions, hematomas, and chronic traumatic encephalopathy are types of TBI that were discussed earlier. Non-accidental trauma occurs when a child younger than five years sustains an injury to the skull or brain because of being shaken or struck by an adult. These types of injuries will often lead to skull fractures and subdural bleeds, among other injuries. Non-accidental trauma has the potential to cause death in children and infants, so patient education, monitoring, and reporting are vital to prevention and survival.

Behavioral/Psychosocial

Agitation

Agitation is an extreme form of arousal associated with increased verbal and motor activity. These symptoms are caused by a variety of etiologies, both medical and psychiatric. Patients with agitation may present not only to an emergency department or a psychiatric emergency service, but also to a clinic or acute care center that does not have the onsite medical resources of a physician or midlevel practitioner. A patient who acts nervous or anxious may be agitated. Agitation in a critically-ill patient, outside the range of normal, may be a sign of underlying mental disturbance.

The Behavioral Activity Rating Scale (BARS), which follows, should be used to assess the severity of agitation.

1. Cannot be roused easily
2. Sleeping, but responsive to verbal and physical contact in a normal fashion
3. Appears drowsy and sedated
4. Normal activity level (quiet and awake)
5. Calms with instructions and shows signs of overt physical or verbal activity
6. Does not require restraints but is continuously or very active
7. Requires restraint because of violence and aggression

Any patient with a BARS score of 1 requires immediate transfer to a medical ED. Patients with a score of 2, 3, or 7 should be transferred immediately to either a medical emergency department or a psychiatric facility with medical capability. For mild to moderate agitation, BARS 5 or 6, the patient may be calmed with verbal de-escalation techniques, and environmental modification. If this is successful, further evaluation at the clinic is acceptable. Oxygenation level and blood sugar level should be obtained if possible. The initial examination should be directed at identifying factors that could indicate serious, possibly life-threatening, conditions. Unless immediate intervention is indicated, de-escalation should be continued to gain patient cooperation.

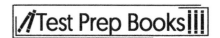

Agitation can be due to a general medical condition, intoxication and withdrawal, or a decompensated psychiatric disease. Drug side effects, a mood disorder such as anxiety or depression, dementia, autism, or a neurological disorder should be ruled out. Finding out the underlying cause of the agitation is key to reversing it. If agitation is caused by a mental health disturbance medication and behavioral therapy may be increased or adjusted to relieve the agitation.

If pharmacological agents are necessary for the treatment of agitation, one of the following three classes will likely be used. First-generation antipsychotics, such as Haldol, work by inhibiting dopamine transmission to the brain, which has a calming effect on the patient. Second-generation antipsychotics, formally called atypical antipsychotics, are serotonin-dopamine antagonists, and are less likely than first-generation antipsychotics to cause extrapyramidal motor control issues. Benzodiazepines act on GABA receptors to reduce anxiety, relax muscles, produce a sedative effect, and can be used as an anticonvulsant. A last resort for a severely agitated patient is the use of physical restraints which require a physician order and must meet strict hospital protocols.

Antisocial Behaviors, Aggression, Violence

People with antisocial personality disorders (ASPD) show no signs of empathy. They have no awareness of how others perceive them, how to interact with others, or how to anticipate their feelings or reactions. To people without empathy, the feelings and emotions of others are not a factor in decision-making, which can lead a spectrum of behaviors that range from social awkwardness to acts of cruelty and negligence. Antisocial actions are what cause many people with antisocial behaviors to break the law or hurt others. There may be a disregard for the truth in pursuit of entertainment or personal gain, usually as a kind of manipulation. Lack of empathy makes it difficult for those with ASPD to contemplate why moral standards constructed for other people are applicable to them. Those with ASPD often lie repeatedly and consistently for personal satisfaction alone.

An aggressive history and a tendency to get into serious fights are an indicator of ASPD, and one that distinguishes it from psychopathy. Aggression is divided into two types, reactive (which comes after a threat), and instrumental (which is for personal gain). Reactive aggression is all about the body's instant reaction to something that seems to be wrong or threatening. It is possible that the brain circuitry of people with ASPD leaps to threatening conclusions much faster than ordinary ones. A 2013 study found that ASPD sufferers were more likely to be reactively aggressive and to have something called hostile intention bias, where they misinterpreted everything as a potential threat.

A study in 2009 found that people with ASPD have very strong rapid-response impulsivity but the same level of impulse control as non-sufferers when it came to future planning. There is a strong need to be independent, to resist being controlled by others, who are usually held in contempt. There is a willingness to use untamed aggression to back up the need for control or independence. The antisocial personality usually presents in a friendly, sociable manner, but that friendliness is always accompanied by a baseline position of detachment. There is a total lack of investment in the comfort of others, a complete focus on their own feelings and complete lack of remorse. It is very common that the person with ASPD is not the one who seeks help; often friends, families, or intimate partners attempt to get a diagnosis.

If the patient is officially diagnosed they may be prescribed cognitive-behavioral therapy, mood stabilizers, and antidepressants. ASPD often comes with accompanying diagnoses of substance abuse disorder, borderline personality disorder, narcissistic personality disorder, and conduct disorder.

Delirium

Delirium is a serious disturbance in mental abilities that results in confused thinking and reduced awareness of the environment. The start of delirium is usually rapid, within hours or a few days. Older people recovering in the hospital or living in a long-term care facility are particularly at risk of delirium. Delirium is a serious disturbance in mental abilities that results in confused thinking and reduced awareness of the environment. People with other serious, chronic or terminal illnesses may not regain the levels of thinking skills or functioning that they had before the onset of delirium.

Delirium occurs when the normal signals in the brain become impaired. Delirium can often be traced to one or more contributing factors, such as a severe or chronic illness, changes in metabolic balance (such as low sodium), medication, infection, surgery, alcohol or drug intoxication, or withdrawal. The most easily recognized type, hyperactive delirium, may include restlessness, pacing, agitation, rapid mood changes or hallucinations, and refusal to cooperate with care. Hypoactive delirium presents as inactivity or reduced motor activity, sluggishness, abnormal drowsiness, or confusion. Mixed delirium includes both hyperactive and hypoactive signs and symptoms. The person may quickly switch back and forth from hyperactive to hypoactive states.

Symptoms often fluctuate throughout the day, and there may be periods of time without symptoms. Delirium becomes worse during the night when things look less familiar in the dark. Delirium may last only a few hours or as long as several weeks or months. If issues contributing to delirium are addressed, the recovery time is often shorter. The degree of recovery depends on the health and mental status before the onset of delirium. The most successful approach to preventing delirium is to target risk factors that might trigger an episode. Hospital environments present a special challenge; frequent room changes, invasive procedures, loud noises, poor lighting, lack of natural light, and sleep can all worsen confusion. Evidence indicates that promoting good sleep habits, remaining calm and oriented, and helping prevent medical complications, can help prevent or reduce the severity of delirium.

Dementia

Dementia is a progressive decline of memory and cognitive skills due to a gradual dysfunction and loss of brain cells. Dementia isn't a specific disease but a description of a group of symptoms affecting memory, thinking and social abilities severely enough to interfere with daily functioning. Depending on the cause, some dementia symptoms can be reversed and having memory loss doesn't mean you have dementia. Alzheimer's disease is the most common cause of a progressive dementia in older adults.

Common symptoms of dementia include:

- Memory loss, which is usually noticed by a spouse or someone else
- Difficulty communicating or finding words
- Difficulty reasoning, problem-solving or handling complex tasks
- Difficulty with planning and organizing
- Difficulty with coordination and motor functions
- Confusion, disorientation, paranoia
- Psychological and personality changes
- Depression, anxiety and inappropriate behavior

Dementia and delirium may be particularly difficult to distinguish, and a person may have both. Delirium frequently occurs in people with dementia, but having episodes of delirium does not always mean a person has dementia. A dementia assessment should not be done during a delirium episode because the results could be misleading. The onset of delirium occurs within a short time, while dementia usually

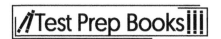

begins with relatively minor symptoms that gradually worsen over time. The ability to stay focused or maintain attention is significantly impaired with delirium whereas a person in the early stages of dementia remains generally alert. The appearance of delirium symptoms can fluctuate significantly and frequently memory and thinking skills stay at a fairly constant level during the course of a day. Patients with dementia often have a significant decline in memory and thinking skills. Because symptoms of delirium and dementia can be similar, input from a family member or caregiver may be important for a doctor to make an accurate diagnosis.

Although the cause of Alzheimer's disease isn't known, plaques and tangles are often found in the brains of people with Alzheimer's. Plaques are clumps of a protein called beta-amyloid, and tangles are fibrous tangles made up of tau protein. Certain genetic factors might make it more likely that people will develop Alzheimer's. It is not reversible.

Vascular dementia is the second most common type of dementia, occurring as a result of damage to the vessels that supply blood to the brain. Abnormal clumps of protein (Lewy Bodies) have been found in the brains of people with dementia, Alzheimer's disease, and Parkinson's disease, all common types of progressive dementia.

Frontotemporal dementia is a group of diseases characterized by the degeneration of nerve cells in the frontal and temporal lobes of the brain, the areas generally associated with personality, behavior and language. The cause isn't known. Autopsy studies of the brains of people 80 and older who had dementia indicate that many had a combination of Alzheimer's disease, vascular dementia and Lewy body dementia. Studies are ongoing to determine how having mixed dementia affects symptoms and treatments. Huntington's disease, a genetic mutation, causes certain nerve cells in the brain and spinal cord to waste away. Signs and symptoms, including a severe decline in cognition, usually appear around age 30 or 40. Traumatic brain injury caused by repetitive head trauma, such as experienced by boxers, football players or soldiers. Has already been discussed. Creutzfeldt-Jakob disease is a rare brain disorder that usually occurs in people without known risk factors. Creutzfeldt-Jakob disease can be inherited or caused by exposure to diseased brain or nervous system tissue. Signs and symptoms of this fatal condition usually appear around age 60.

Some causes of dementia or dementia-like symptoms can be reversed with treatment. They include: infections and immune disorders; Metabolic problems and endocrine abnormalities; nutritional deficiencies; reactions to medications; subdural hematomas; exposure to heavy metals; and anoxia. Some factors, such as age, can't be changed, while others can be addressed to reduce risk. The symptoms of depression may mimic dementia and depression may be the first sign of dementia. It is estimated that up to forty percent of those diagnosed with Alzheimer's also have significant cases of depression.

As the disease progresses, the patient may become increasingly agitated and uncooperative, in some cases even physically aggressive. The patient may hallucinate, become delusional, and feel persecuted and paranoid. At this point their sleep patterns have become interrupted or erratic. By the late stage of dementia, the activities that the patient does daily become a challenge, such as controlling their bowels and bladder, getting dressed, feeding themselves, and so on. They become unable to report their own symptoms if they are ill. Infection is the leading cause of death in these individuals, related to their inability to communicate symptoms. Because this condition is irreversible, symptom management and supportive care are the mainstay treatments, ensuring the highest quality of life for as long as possible.

Medical Non-Adherence

Medical non-adherence can refer to patients not taking their medication appropriately or not following the recommendations and prescribed treatments. Each individual patient case is different and each case of non-adherence must be addressed based on patient circumstances and needs.

Medication nonadherence is widely recognized as a common and costly problem. Approximately 30% to 50% of US adults are not adherent to long-term medications. This leads to an estimated $100 billion in preventable costs in healthcare annually. Despite the widespread prevalence and cost of medication nonadherence, it is undetected and undertreated in a significant proportion of adults across care settings. The World Health Organization estimates that increasing the effectiveness of adherence may have a greater impact on the health of the population than any improvement in specific medical treatments.

One way to identify the population of at risk for medication non-adherence is to conduct screenings. However, most clinicians are not formally trained on screening for, and diagnosing, medication nonadherence, nor are they fully aware of how best to treat nonadherence if detected. One of the most common diagnostic assessments for medication nonadherence is simply asking patients if they have any problems taking the medication regimen as prescribed When no further questions are asked, potentially addressable medication issues are left unattended.

Mood Disorders, Depression, Anxiety

A mood disorder is a mental health class that broadly describe all types of depression and bipolar disorders. The following are the most common types of mood disorders:

1. Major depression: having less interest in usual activities, feeling sad or hopeless, and other symptoms for at least 2 weeks.

2. Dysthymia: a chronic, low-grade, depressed, or irritable mood that lasts for at least 2 years.

3. Bipolar disorder: a condition in which a person has periods of depression alternating with periods of mania or elevated mood.

4. Mood disorder related to another health condition: having an acute or chronic medical illnesses can trigger symptoms of depression.

5. Substance-induced mood disorder: symptoms of depression that are due to the effects of medicine, drug abuse, alcoholism, exposure to toxins, or other forms of treatment.

Mood disorders may be caused by an imbalance of brain chemicals. Life events, abrupt changes in routine, and stress may also contribute to a depressed mood. Mood disorders also tend to run in families and are more intense and harder to manage than normal feelings of sadness. Children, teens, or adults who have a parent with a mood disorder have a greater chance of also having a mood disorder. Rates of depression are nearly twice as high as in women as they are in men. Once a person in the family has this diagnosis, their brothers, sisters, or children have a higher chance of the same diagnosis. Depending on age and the type of mood disorder, a person may have different symptoms of depression. The following are the most common symptoms of a mood disorder:

- Ongoing sad, anxious, or empty affect
- Feeling hopeless or helpless
- Having low self-esteem

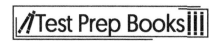

- Feeling inadequate or worthless
- Excessive guilt
- Repeating thoughts of death or suicide
- Loss of interest in usual activities or activities that were once enjoyed, including sex
- Relationship problems
- Trouble sleeping or sleeping too much
- Changes in appetite and/or weight
- Decreased energy
- Trouble concentrating
- A decrease in the ability to make decisions
- Frequent physical complaints that don't get better with treatment
- Very sensitive to failure or rejection
- Irritability, hostility, or aggression

With a mood disorders, these feelings are more intense than what a person may feel occasionally. If these feelings continue over time, interfere with interest in family, friends, community, or work, or if there are thoughts of suicide, medical intervention is needed.

Antidepressant and mood stabilizing medicines, especially when combined with psychotherapy, have been shown to work very well in the treatment of depression. Treatment of bipolar disorder may include mood stabilizers such as lithium and carbamazepine, along with second-generation antipsychotics such as aripiprazole and risperidone. Psychotherapy is focused on changing the person's distorted views of self and the environment. It also helps to improve interpersonal relationship skills, identify stressors in the environment, and assist with avoiding them. Family therapy, electroconvulsive therapy, and transcranial stimulation may also be therapeutic.

Post-Traumatic Stress Disorder (PTSD)

PTSD is a disorder that develops in some people who have experienced a shocking, scary, or dangerous event. People who have PTSD may feel stressed or frightened even when they are not in danger. Fear triggers many split-second changes in the body to help defend against danger or to avoid it. This fight-or-flight response is a typical reaction meant to protect a person from harm. Most people recover from initial symptoms naturally but those who continue to be diagnosed with PTSD.

Symptoms usually begin within 3 months of the traumatic incident, but may occur later. Symptoms must last more than a month and be severe enough to interfere with relationships or work to be considered PTSD. The course of the illness varies, and it may become chronic. Some people recover within 6 months, while others have symptoms that last much longer. Re-experiencing symptoms may cause problems in a person's everyday routine. The symptoms can start from the person's own thoughts and feelings. Words, objects, or situations that are reminders of the event can also trigger re-experiencing symptoms.

To be diagnosed with PTSD, an adult must have all of the following for at least 1 month:

- At least one re-experiencing symptom
- At least one avoidance symptom
- At least two arousal and reactivity symptoms
- At least two cognition and mood symptoms
- Re-experiencing symptoms include:

- Flashbacks—reliving the trauma over and over, including physical symptoms like a racing heart or sweating
- Bad dreams
- Frightening thoughts

Avoidance symptoms include staying away from places, events, or objects that are reminders of the traumatic experience and avoiding thoughts or feelings related to the traumatic event. Things that remind a person of the traumatic event can trigger avoidance symptoms. These symptoms may cause a person to change his or her personal routine. For example, after a bad car accident, a person who usually drives may avoid driving or riding in a car.

Arousal and reactivity symptoms include: being easily startled, feeling tense, having difficulty sleeping, and having angry outbursts. Arousal symptoms are usually constant, instead of being triggered by things that remind one of the traumatic events. These symptoms can make the person feel stressed and angry. They may make it hard to do daily tasks, such as sleeping, eating, or concentrating.

Cognition and mood symptoms include: trouble remembering key features of the traumatic event, negative thoughts about self or the world, distorted feelings like guilt or blame, and loss of interest in enjoyable activities. Cognition and mood symptoms can begin or worsen after the traumatic event, but are not due to injury or substance use. These symptoms can make the person feel alienated or detached from friends or family members.

Anyone can develop PTSD at any age. This includes war veterans, children, and people who have been through a physical or sexual assault, abuse, accident, disaster, or many other serious events. According to the National Center for PTSD, about 7 or 8 out of every 100 people will experience PTSD at some point in their lives. Women are more likely to develop PTSD than men, and genes may make some people more likely to develop PTSD than others.

The main treatments for people with PTSD are medications, psychotherapy, or both. Everyone is different, and PTSD affects people differently so a treatment that works for one person may not work for another. It is important for anyone with PTSD to be treated by a mental health provider who is experienced with PTSD. Some people with PTSD need to try different treatments to find what works for their symptoms. As genetic research and brain imaging technologies continue to improve, scientists are more likely to be able to pinpoint when and where in the brain PTSD begins. This understanding may then lead to better targeted treatments to suit each person's own needs or even prevent the disorder before it causes harm.

A 2012 study of 395 military veterans with PTSD found a link between risk-taking behavior and the disorder. In addition to the above forms of riskiness, vets with PTSD have a propensity for firearms play, potentially endangering their lives. People with PTSD have already survived dangerous situations and risk-taking behavior may give such individuals the feeling that they have more control over their present circumstances than those that led to them developing PTSD. Recognizing this propensity in their personality may help patients with risk-taking behavior, thus being the first step in remediating the problem. Behavioral and cognitive therapy, as well as psychological drugs such as antidepressants, may also aid in the treatment of this behavior.

Risk-Taking Behavior

Risk-taking behaviors such as driving fast or engaging in substance use, may lead to car accidents or overdoses, respectively. Yet, they may bring about positive feelings in the moment. This includes the thrill of a fast ride or the high one gets from drug use. Given that risk-taking behavior is potentially dangerous, some people wonder why anyone would take part in such conduct. On one hand, such behavior puts those who engage in it in harm's way, but, on the other, it gives participants the chance to experience an outcome they perceive as positive. Sigmund Freud theorized that this was related to an innate drive within human beings to seek experiences that put them close to death, for the adrenaline high one might feel. Risk-taking behavior can be a singular diagnosis or it can be part of the symptomology of other conditions such as PTSD.

Risk-taking behavior includes having sex with strangers, often with no protection against sexually transmitted diseases or unplanned pregnancies. Risk-takers also enjoy gambling, typically losing more than they can handle. These individuals may also take part in extreme sports or recreational activities.

Some research indicates that men tend to be more likely to be risk-takers than women. But both male and female risk-takers share the same personality traits, such as impulsive sensation-seeking, aggression-hostility, and sociability, one study found. Genetics play a role in risk-taking behavior and identical twins separated at birth, for example, tend to engage in risk-taking behaviors at high rates. Testosterone appears to play a role as well, which is why there's a gender imbalance in the people most likely to take part in risk-taking behaviors.

Substance Dependence or Abuse

In 2013, the American Psychological Association (APA) released the fifth edition of the DSM. In this edition, the definitions revolving around addiction were changed. The APA threw away both "substance abuse" and "substance dependence" in favor of "substance use disorder." The difference between addiction and dependence can be difficult to understand. Some organizations have different definitions, use the words interchangeably or even abandon both terms altogether.

The term dependence usually refers to a physical dependence on a substance, characterized by tolerance and withdrawal. While it is possible to have a physical dependence without being addicted, addiction is usually right around the corner. Addiction is marked by a change in behavior caused by the biochemical changes in the brain after continued substance abuse. Substance use becomes the main priority of the addict, regardless of the harm they may cause to themselves or others. An addiction causes people to act irrationally when they don't have the substance they are addicted to in their system. Addiction encompasses both a mental and physical reliance on a given substance.

When the symptoms of mental and physical dependence are apparent, an addiction is usually present. However, the main characteristic that distinguishes addiction from dependence is the combination of mental and physical dependence with uncontrollable behavior in obtaining and using a substance. Triggers can be emotional responses to events, certain people, places or anything a person associates with using a substance.

Abuse and dependence are defined on a scale that measures the time and degree of substance use. Essentially, abuse is like the early stage of dependence. As substance abuse becomes more frequent, the likelihood of developing a dependence disorder becomes greater.

Suicidal Ideation and/or Behaviors

It is important to take people seriously when they express having suicidal thoughts. Research has shown that about one-fifth of people who die by suicide had talked to their doctor or other healthcare professional about their decision. These types of thoughts may arise in people who feel completely hopeless or believe they can no longer cope with their life situation. Suicidal ideation can vary greatly from fleeting thoughts to preoccupation to detailed planning.

According to the CDC, for every 25 attempts, there is one suicide death, Suicide is the tenth leading cause of death for all ages in the United States, and the third leading cause of death among 15 to 24 year-olds. Patients with borderline personality disorder face an extraordinarily high risk of suicidal ideation and suicide attempts. One study showed that 73% of patients with borderline personality disorder have attempted suicide, with the average patient having 3.4 attempts.

Warning signs may include hopelessness, racing thoughts, insomnia or oversleeping, mania, loss of appetite or overeating, loneliness, alcohol abuse, excessive fatigue or low self-esteem. Research has found a variety of risk factors for suicidal ideation including the following:

- Mood and mental disorders
- Adverse life or family events (divorce, death of a loved one, job loss)
- Chronic illness or pain
- Previous suicide attempt
- Military experience
- Witnessing trauma
- Family violence
- Owning a gun
- Being the victim of abuse or bullying
- Unplanned pregnancy
- Drug or alcohol abuse

An act that is intended to cause injury but not death is called a non-suicidal self-injury. An example of this type of behavior is when patients cut themselves. It is a method of relieving psychological pain through physical pain. Men are more likely than women to commit suicide, as well as more likely to abuse alcohol and drugs concurrently. Men are less likely to seek help when they are depressed. Veterans have seen an increase in suicides in recent years. It is important to note that despite these risk factors for suicide, it can occur across a wide span of age groups, genders, and life circumstances.

Some patients who are more vocal about their suicidal ideation may be crying out for help and must be taken very seriously. Treatment should include psychotherapy and antidepressants. It should be noted, however, that antidepressants sometimes have the adverse side effect of worsened suicidal behavior. Caregivers should be instructed to be watchful for deepening of depression and thus an increased risk for suicide. Suicide hotlines are available to help suicidal patients in moments of crisis.

Multisystem

Bariatric Complications

Bariatric surgery is increasingly being performed in the medically complicated obese population as convincing data continue to mount, documenting the success of surgery not only in achieving meaningful weight loss but also in correcting obesity-related illnesses. The 4 most common bariatric

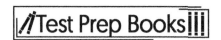

surgical procedures are: laparoscopic adjustable gastric banding, vertical sleeve gastrectomy, Roux-en-Y gastric bypass, and biliopancreatic diversion with duodenal switch.

Bariatric surgery is increasingly being accepted as a viable treatment for managing the growing obesity epidemic. Surgery can provide a sustainable, long-term option for weight loss. The prevalence of obesity (body mass index [BMI] ≥30 kg/m2) has stabilized at 35% in the United States since 2003. However, it is estimated that only 1% of eligible patients are undergoing surgical intervention. One barrier to accepting surgery may be the false notion of unacceptable risks and high rate of complications associated with surgery.

Obesity is associated with multiple medical comorbidities, including type 2 diabetes mellitus, cardiovascular disease, dyslipidemia, hypertension, cholelithiasis, gastroesophageal reflux disease, obstructive sleep apnea, degenerative joint disease, lower back pain, and cancer. In addition, obesity is associated with an increase in early mortality. The estimated number of annual deaths attributed to obesity in US adults is 280,000.

In 1991, the National Institutes of Health consensus panel developed a set of recommendations regarding which patients should be considered for bariatric surgery. These recommendations included the criteria that patients have a calculated BMI of at least 40 kg/m2 or a BMI of at least 35 kg/m2 with significant obesity-related comorbidities. Along with the increased volume of surgical procedures, a dramatic decrease in mortality and complications related to surgical intervention has been achieved, as demonstrated in a recent meta-analysis showing a mortality rate of 0.08% within 30 days and 0.31% after 30 days. Complication rates from bariatric operations have progressively fallen from 10.5% of cases in 1993 to 7.6% of cases in 2006, with the majority of complications now being minor.

Comorbidity in Patients with Transplant History

It is common to have some medical problems after transplant. Many transplant recipients manage two or more diseases at the same time. Some of the most common are: Cancer, diabetes, hypertension, kidney disease, and cardiovascular disease.

Cancer is more common in transplant patients than the general population. Research has shown that it is likely for patients who live for at least 10 years after a transplant to develop some type of cancer, including skin cancer. The main risk factors contributing to an increased incidence of any cancer is due to suppression of the immune system, and duration and intensity of immunosuppression. All types of immunosuppressant medications can increase the risk for certain types of cancer.

The best option for improving outcomes in transplant recipients is to stabilize and improve any existing comorbidities as much as possible before performing the operation. This will, in turn, improve the probability of the transplant tissue being accepted. Obesity is one example of a comorbidity that often complicates outcomes, including transplant tissue acceptance or rejection. Improving diet and maintaining regular exercise programs, as well as correcting obesity-related behaviors such as binge-eating, may improve the probability of transplant acceptance.

Graft-vs-host disease (GVHD) may occur as a comorbidity of transplantation. This may manifest itself as fever, rash, hepatitis, vomiting, diarrhea, and abdominal pain. Patients who are unrelated to the tissue donor or are of older age may be at greater risk for developing GVHD, which may be acute or chronic. Prevention of GVHD includes more accurate screening methods for matching donor and recipient. Treatment of GVHD may include methylprednisolone IV as an immunosuppressant while the transplant tissue heals.

End of Life

Nurses provide comprehensive and compassionate end-of-life care. This includes recognizing when death is near and conveying that information to families. Nurses should collaborate with other members of the health care team to ensure optimal symptom management and to provide support for the patient and family.

Nurses and other health care providers have a responsibility to establish decision-making processes that reflect physiologic realities, patient preferences, and the recognition of what, clinically, may or may not be accomplished. Establishing goals of care for this patient at this time may provide a framework for discussion about what care should be provided. This process often involves collaboration with experts in decision-making, such as ethics committees or palliative care teams. Decision-making for the end of a patient's life should occur over years rather than just in the minutes or days before a patient's death. Nurses can be a resource and support for patients and families at the end of a patient's life and in the decision-making process that precedes it. Nurses are often ideally positioned to contribute to conversations about end-of-life care and decisions, including maintaining a focus on patient preferences, and to establish mechanisms to respect the patient's autonomy.

There are times when the preferences of the family do not represent, or are in conflict with, the preferences of the patient. In those cases, the nurse's primary responsibility is to provide care and support to the patient and to respect the patient's autonomy while continuing to support the family as they struggle to adjust to the impending reality of the patient's death. Standards for excellent care for patients at the end of life should be evidence based, and should integrate national and international standards of care.

Nursing care includes not only disease management but also attention to physical comfort, and the recognition that patient well-being also includes psychological, interpersonal, and spiritual dimensions. Nurses have the knowledge and skills to manage pain and other distressing symptoms for patients with serious or life-limiting illness, and to work with patients and their families in palliative and end-of-life care decision-making.

Advance directives are an expression of the patient's preferences for medical care that are based on a person's values and beliefs. Advance directives come into play when that person is unable to, or chooses not to make decisions. Advance directives include identification of a surrogate, someone who will represent the patient's preferences in decision-making. Examples of advance directives include durable powers of attorney for health care, do not resuscitate order, and medical/physician orders for life-sustaining therapy (MOLST, POLST).

The loved ones of the dying patient need support as well. Educating them on what to expect when their loved one passes will help them be ready for the moment. The patient will likely lose consciousness and the ability to speak in the final days and hours. When the patient does pass, bereavement services should be made available to the surviving loved ones. Cultural preferences should be honored. Quiet time alone with the body may be desired and this request should be respected. Many hospitals have designated rooms and floors for end-of-life care, and spaces for the bereaved to mourn. Proper, dignified end-of-life care by the nurse and the healthcare team will aid in the healing process for the loved ones who remain.

Healthcare-Associated Infections (HAI)

Due to the invasive nature of caring for a patient, there is almost always a risk for infection when a patient enters the healthcare environment. From IV lines and urinary catheters to ventilators, there are many different ways that the immune system can become compromised.

Central Line-Associated Bloodstream Infections (CLABSI)

Many patients who are critically ill will need a central venous catheter. These central lines are often placed in the neck, groin, or chest of the patient for access to large blood vessels. The larger the vessel, the more medications, fluid, and blood transfusions can be administered to quickly stabilize critically ill patients. The problem with these lines, as with any other route into a body that does not naturally occur, is that they are prone to infection. Infection not only complicates the patient's care, but it also worsens the patient's chance of making a fast and full recovery from the original illness.

The critical care nurse must be extremely cautious when placing, caring for, and removing central lines, to prevent infectious agents from entering the patient's body. Hand hygiene is the first line of defense. When assisting with the placement of the central line, the nurse must don sterile gloves, gown, cap, mask, and utilize proper sterile draping. After placement, the nurse must strictly follow maintenance practices such as dressing changes as outlined by the facility. To prevent infection, the central line must be removed as soon as it is no longer needed.

Central line-associated bloodstream infection (CLABSI) and catheter-associated urinary tract infection (CAUTI) are costly and morbid. Despite evidence-based guidelines, some ICUs continue to have elevated infection rates.

Catheter-Associated Urinary Tract Infection (CAUTI)

Patients admitted to the critical care unit will often have urinary catheters for collecting, measuring, and observing urine output. Some patients may be at risk for skin breakdown that is aggravated by urinary incontinence and have a catheter for that reason. Whatever the reason for the urinary catheter, the nurse must be aware of its potential for causing infection and take steps to prevent such infections. Hand hygiene before and after caring for the patient is always one of the best ways to prevent the spread of infection. The nurse must ensure that aseptic technique is practiced when placing the urinary catheter. As with the central line, the urinary catheter must be removed as soon as it is no longer needed. Most hospitals have strict policies and procedures in place to prevent catheter-associated urinary tract infections (CAUTIs). They usually have checklists that must be addressed before placing the catheter, and daily while the patient has it. When the patient no longer meets criteria for having a catheter, the catheter must be removed to prevent infection.

VAP (Ventilator-Associated Event or VAE)

Patients who are on mechanical ventilation are at risk of developing a lung infection related to being intubated, referred to as **ventilator-associated pneumonia** or VAP. The endotracheal tube used in mechanical ventilation is a foreign body in the airway, one that poses risk of infection. Microorganisms can easily use the tube as a route of entry to the patient's lungs; thus, special care must be given to prevent these types of infections.

The first and foremost way VAP may be prevented is limiting the amount of time the patient is on mechanical ventilation. The sooner that foreign object can be removed from the airway, the better. Hand hygiene for general care and sterile technique for invasive procedures are vital prevention techniques. Raising the head of the patient's bed to at least 45 degrees may aid in preventing bacteria from traveling down the tube and into the patient's lungs. Some hospitals use antiseptic mouthwashes such as chlorhexidine to keep the patient's oral cavity clean, thus preventing bacterial and other infectious growths from occurring.

Hypotension

Hypotension is a blood pressure reading below 90 mmHg systolic side and below 60 mmHg diastolic. The patient's blood pressure could be low, due to low circulating volume, too many hypertensive medications, central nervous system depression, or heart failure. Determining the underlying cause of the hypotension will aid in correcting it.

Postural hypotension occurs when the pressure drops because the patient changes positions from sitting to standing. This is often rooted in cardiovascular or neurological disease, in which one of these systems fails to compensate for the change in body position. If low circulating volume is the culprit, fluid volume resuscitation should correct it. If it is postural hypotension, repositioning the patient so that they are lying flat may be the first step in correcting the low blood pressure. When hypotension occurs, blood flow is reduced and the result is decreased perfusion of the organs, thereby reducing their functioning. IV medications such as dopamine, dobutamine, or norepinephrine may be infused to raise the pressure.

Infectious Diseases

Multidrug-Resistant Organisms

Over time, due to overuse of antibiotics, some organisms have become resistant to treatments that used to work. They have mutated in such a way that they can no longer be killed with previously effective antibiotics. Methicillin-resistant staphylococcus aureus (MRSA) is one such organism. Sometimes called a super bug, it is highly resistant to common antibiotic treatments. Discovered in the 1960s when it was resistant only to methicillin, it is now resistant to amoxicillin, penicillin, and oxacillin. MRSA infections spread by contact and are common in those with weakened immune systems who are admitted to healthcare facilities. Catheters, central lines, and surgical wounds are common sites for MRSA infections.

Vancomycin-resistant enterococci (VRE) and carbapenem-resistant Enterobacteriaceae (CRE) follow the same pattern as MRSA. VRE and CRE have become resistant to vancomycin and carbapenem, respectively, and are increasingly difficult to treat, as they continue to mutate. Both VRE and CRE are like MRSA in that they most commonly affect patients with weakened immune systems in healthcare settings. All three occur around central lines, ventilators, and urinary catheters.

Treating drug-resistant organisms can be tough, but not impossible. An intensive regimen of antibiotics that will kill the specific infection is necessary. Prevention is always the best intervention; practice meticulous handwashing, contact precautions, and remove lines as early as possible held reduce the spread of drug-resistant infections.

Influenza

Influenza is a type of virus that causes an upper respiratory infection of three types (A, B, and C). Some infections are mistakenly called the "flu," but are not actually caused by the influenza virus, resulting in a bit of confusion. A nasal swab can differentiate between influenza and other organisms. Symptoms of the flu include cough, coryza, fever, headache, and a generalized malaise. Flu season differs around the world, occurring in the coldest months of the year when the flu virus thrives. In the US, the accepted season is October through March. The number of influenza infections in a geographic region sometimes escalates rapidly, turning into an epidemic.

Everyone over 6 months of age should be vaccinated against the flu annually, at the beginning of their respective flu season. Patients at high risk of developing a severe case of influenza infection may be given antivirals. Those at lower risk may be treated for symptoms alone, allowing the virus to run its course naturally.

When influenza occurs at the pandemic level it may be severe enough to cause even healthy, young patients to die. For this reason, vaccination of the population is vital.

Multi-Organ Dysfunction Syndrome (MODS)

The incremental process by which multiple organs start shutting down individually is called multiple organ dysfunction syndrome (MODS). It is a process rather than a single event and may take place slowly over the course of days to weeks. Alteration in organ function can vary widely from a mild degree of organ dysfunction to completely irreversible organ failure. The degree of organ dysfunction has a major clinical impact. Failure of these multiple organ systems may or may not be related to the initial injury or disease process for which the patient was admitted to the ICU.

MODS is the leading cause of morbidity and mortality in current ICU practice. While the pathophysiology of MODS is not completely known, much evidence indicates that, during the initial injury which precipitates ICU admission, a chain of events is initiated which results in activation of several metabolic pathways. These pathways release compounds which results in an inflammatory response which can lead to development of failure in distant organs. As these organs fail, they activate and propagate the systemic inflammatory response. No therapy has proven successful at reducing the response or the incidence and severity of MODS. Treatment is focused on prevention and treating individual organ dysfunction as it develops. investigation.

Multisystem Trauma

To improve survival in the patient with multiple injuries, the injuries are prioritized. The order of priority among injuries is related to time and degree of life threat posed by each injury. Immediate priority is given to airway control and to maintenance of ventilation, oxygenation, and perfusion. Complete in-depth assessment of the multiply injured patient is required only after immediately life-threatening injuries have been treated. Then, repeated assessment is necessary to diagnose and treat injuries that are not obvious on initial presentation.

Death occurring at the scene results from such injuries as cardiac rupture or disruption of the major intrathoracic vessels, and severe brain injury that is incompatible with survival. In these cases, death occurs within minutes of the traumatic event and medical intervention is usually futile. The second peak in mortality following multiple injuries occurs from minutes to a few hours after the event. Mortality during this phase is related to injuries that are immediately life-threatening, such as airway compromise, tension pneumothorax, and cardiac tamponade. This is also a period during which simple appropriate resuscitative measures can significantly affect the outcome. The third peak occurs as a result of complications of the injury, such as sepsis or multiple-system organ failure. Mortality in this third phase can be affected by the type of intervention during the second phase.

Blunt trauma from motor vehicle collision is the most frequent cause of injuries in general. This type of impact usually results in injuries to many different parts of the body simultaneously. The healthcare team must be prepared to deal with multisystem traumas with several teams ready to receive, stabilize, and care for the patient. Gunshot wounds, car crash injuries, penetrating wounds from knives, and being punched and kicked repeatedly will all result in multiple systems of the body being traumatized.

When a multisystem trauma patient is received in the field, the emergency team will work to stop bleeding, stabilize the cervical spine, and maintain a patent airway. Once the patient arrives at the hospital, they may be immediately transported to the surgical suite for stabilization of the internal bleeding. Once internal bleeding is stopped, repair can be made to any remaining tears, perforations, or other injuries sustained. The critical care nurse assists with many of these interventions along the patient's care path. Hemodynamic monitoring is ongoing. Fluid resuscitation and blood transfusions are necessary for patients who have experienced massive bleeding. The nurse must be cognizant of signs that the patient's condition may be worsening, such as the development of a fever, dropping or rising blood pressure, or changes in heart rate. Once stabilization has been achieved, care must be taken to prevent infection around open wounds and central lines. Maintaining clean dressings, performing meticulous hand hygiene, and observing proper precautions for the individual patient will all help prevent infections.

Pain

Pain has been called the fifth vital sign and is an important clue as to how well the patient is doing. Pain is the most frequent reason patients seek medical care. Pain has sensory and emotional components and is classified as acute or chronic. Acute pain is frequently associated with anxiety and hyperactivity of the sympathetic nervous system (tachycardia, increased respiratory rate and BP, diaphoresis, dilated pupils). Chronic pain does not involve sympathetic hyperactivity, but may be associated with vegetative signs and depressed mood.

People vary considerably in their tolerance for pain. However, the severity of tissue injury does not always predict the severity of chronic or acute pain. Chronic pain may also result from ongoing damage to or dysfunction of the peripheral or central nervous system, which then causes neuropathic pain.

Somatic pain receptors are located in skin, subcutaneous tissues, fascia, other connective tissues, periosteum, endosteum, and joint capsules. Stimulation of these receptors usually produces sharp or dull localized pain, but burning is not uncommon if the skin or subcutaneous tissues are involved. Visceral pain receptors are located in most viscera and the surrounding connective tissue. Visceral pain due to obstruction of a hollow organ is poorly localized, deep, and cramping and may be referred to remote cutaneous sites. Visceral pain due to injury of organs or other deep connective tissues may be more localized and sharp.

Thoughts and emotions have an important role in the perception of pain. Many patients who have chronic pain also have psychologic distress, especially depression and anxiety. Because certain syndromes characterized as psychiatric are defined by self-reported pain, patients with poorly explained pain are often mischaracterized as having a psychiatric disorder and are thus deprived of appropriate care. Pain impairs attention, memory, concentration, and content of thought.

The common measure of pain is the pain scale, rated one to ten. The nurse assess pain by asking the patient what aggravates the pain, alleviates it, the location, quality, and onset. The nurse should ask about when exacerbations occur, what signs and symptoms accompany an exacerbation, how the pain affects overall functioning ability, how intense it becomes, and its temporal characteristics.

A simple tool to determine what type of medication is helpful for different pain levels is the World Health Organization ladder:

- Step 1. Mild pain (intensity 1 to 3): acetaminophen; NSAIDS; adjuvant medications, such as tricyclic antidepressants and muscle relaxants

- Step 2. Moderate pain (4 to 6 intensity): combination opioids, such as hydrocodone and acetaminophen or oxycodone and acetaminophen, plus continued adjuvant drugs

- Step 3. Severe pain (7 to 10 intensity): opioids, such as morphine and hydromorphone, plus continued adjuvant drugs.

Palliative Care

With patients who are at the end of life (EOL), curative options are discontinued, except those that relieve symptoms such as palliative chemotherapy. Palliative care provides aggressive symptom management, supported decision-making, and end-of-life care. In many cases palliative care isn't introduced until the patient reaches the brink of death. Many patients and healthcare providers aren't aware palliative care can ease symptoms and mistakenly assume it is the same thing as hospice care. Although palliative care was recognized as a specialty in 2006, there are still relatively few specially-trained practitioners.

When a patient nears death, the goal of care changes from cure to comfort, and relieving symptoms is one of the most valuable contributions healthcare professionals can offer. Palliative care practitioners also can help families make difficult decisions on such issues as the patient's code status or whether to use a feeding tube.

Early intervention with palliative care can lead to a better quality of life, improved sleep, less fatigue, and decreased pain, all which enhance the patient's sense of well-being. Primary palliative care refers to the knowledge and skills of palliative care that all providers should have, including basic symptom management, the ability to support decision-making, and the ability to provide support for patients and families. Specialist palliative care refers to the use of consultant specialists with expert knowledge in palliative care to improve care of patients and families. This is much the same model as is used to enhance cardiovascular, renal, neurologic, or other dimensions of patient care.

Discussing the goals of care gives healthcare providers a sense of how the family feels about specific therapies and clarifies questions or misperceptions. Family members might be unfamiliar with the decisions that need to be made, so they must be educated to ensure they fully understand the options. Taking the time to teach them about the benefits of pain relief can make them more comfortable with treatment. The day a person dies should be as important as the day of birth. Each patient is a unique individual and should be celebrated.

Pain is the most common EOL symptom. Approximately 75% of patients with advanced cancer experience pain. No matter what the cause, pain relief is a top priority because it can improve quality of life and relieve stress. Significant pain calls for aggressive pain management, including both pharmacologic and nonpharmacologic options as needed. Many dying patients experience pain for long periods even before reaching EOL. Morphine and hydromorphone commonly are used for pain relief at EOL. If the patient is still able to take oral medication, rapid dose escalation may be needed, with liberal doses given for breakthrough pain (such as incident pain or end-of-dose failure). Extended-release forms of morphine, oxycodone, and hydromorphone can provide a baseline for pain relief, with short-acting opioids used for breakthrough pain. If the patient is able to activate PCA pump with a continuous infusion and patient-activated boluses, a portable pump can be provided for both home and hospital use. Opioids commonly used in PCA pumps include morphine, hydromorphone, and fentanyl citrate. An epidural catheter can provide excellent pain relief using a solution of a local anesthetic and an opioid. The epidural catheter can remain in use for up to 30 days; it's replaced for another 30 days if needed.

Rhabdomyolysis

A breakdown of the skeletal muscle that causes the release of muscle contents into the bloodstream is called rhabdomyolysis. Myoglobin is the skeletal muscle content that is leaked and can be detected in elevated levels in the urine. Diagnosis is made based on symptoms and urinalysis. Rhabdomyolysis may occur for many different reasons, any of which include an insult to the muscle tissue that causes its breakdown. Among the common reasons for the development of rhabdomyolysis are crush injuries, severe burns, cocaine use with hyperthermia, extreme physical activity such as heavy eccentric weight training or marathon training, drug and/or alcohol intoxication, a prolonged comatose state, falls in the elderly followed by prolonged lying on the ground, and prolonged seizures.

A patient with rhabdomyolysis may be asymptomatic. If symptoms do present, they may include muscle pain or myalgia, stiffness, and weakness. The patient's urine may become a dark amber, resembling the color of cola. Rhabdomyolysis may progress quickly to kidney failure. The kidneys have trouble processing myoglobin and begin to shut down as a result. Rhabdomyolysis may also lead to compartment syndrome, where muscle swelling and rising pressure within a confined space compromises the blood circulation to the area. The lower leg is often the site of compartment syndrome.

Treatment of rhabdomyolysis depends on the underlying cause. IV fluid resuscitation will likely be used to flush out the toxic muscle contents and prevent further damage. Electrolytes may be replaced if they are imbalanced. If there is underlying muscle disease, this must be treated. The case is much more complicated if kidney failure has occurred, making early detection crucial to preventing damage to the kidneys.

Sepsis Continuum

In the case of systemic inflammatory response syndrome, or SIRS, two or more criteria must be met: a temperature of greater than 38 degrees Celsius or less than 36 degrees Celsius; a pulse of greater than 90 beats per minute; a respiratory rate of greater than 20 breaths per minute; or a white blood cell count of greater than 12,000. Two or more of these criteria being met in a critically ill patient would suggest that a systemic inflammatory response has begun and potential complications may be ahead. SIRS is the first step in a continuum of worsening illness.

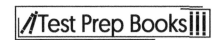

The next stage after SIRS is sepsis, in which criteria for SIRS has been met and there is a known source of infection. Severe sepsis follows when sepsis is present along with organ dysfunction and/or hypotensive crisis. Septic shock occurs when severe sepsis is present, hypotension is unresponsive to fluid resuscitation, and hypoperfusion abnormalities are present. Lactic acidosis, oliguria, and altered mental status are examples of hypoperfusion abnormalities. Multiple organ dysfunction syndrome, or MODS, is the final step in the continuum, with evidence of more than two organs failing. Treatment of the continuum of SIRS to MODS includes fluid resuscitation, blood cultures to identify the source of infection, empirical antibiotics to fight infection, vasopressors for hypotensive support, lactate level measurements, and central venous pressure measurement.

The Sepsis Continuum

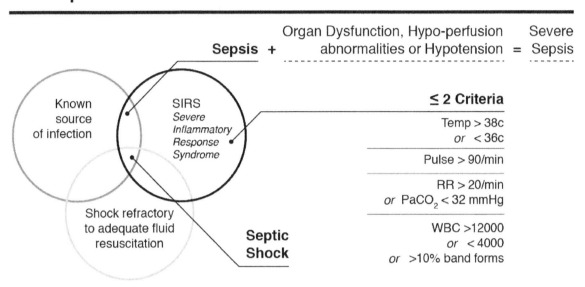

Shock States
Shock occurs in the body when the blood pressure suddenly falls and perfusion is lost to the vital organs. Shock patients will often present with tachycardia, tachypnea, hypotension, altered mental status, and oliguria.

Distributive
Distributive shock is a type of hypotensive crisis in which the vascular smooth muscle is no longer vasoconstricting but massively vasodilating, resulting in dropped pressures systemically. The vascular bed is not responsive to vasoconstrictive agents. Fluid resuscitation may be occurring, but hypotension persists with mixed venous oxygen saturations. This type of shock may occur because of an anaphylactic response in the body after exposure to an allergen. An injury to the brain or spinal cord may also result in distributive shock, referred to as neurogenic.

To treat distributive shock, an ICU admission is necessary. Constant hemodynamic monitoring, measurement of intake and output, respiratory support, and possible endotracheal intubation are all types of intervention for stabilizing the patient. Discovering the underlying cause of distributive shock and reversing it is a priority.

Hypovolemic

Patients who are dehydrated or have lost massive amounts of blood from injury may progress into hypovolemic shock. If bleeding is the cause, it must be stopped as soon as possible. Concurrent with efforts to stop hemorrhaging, fluid resuscitation is performed to raise the patient's blood pressure and bring vital oxygen to the organs and tissues of the body.

Losing more than twenty percent of the body's total blood volume is considered life threatening and will likely throw the body into hypovolemic shock. Organ failure will follow profound hypotension as the heart struggles to compensate for the blood loss. Conditions that may dehydrate the body and cause a significant loss of blood volume include severe burns, prolonged diarrhea, excessive vomiting, and excessive sweating. Treatment for hypovolemic shock will be correction of underlying cause, vasoactive drugs, and most importantly, fluid resuscitation.

Sleep Disruptions

Critically-ill patients frequently experience poor sleep, characterized by frequent disruptions, loss of circadian rhythms, and a lack of time spent in restorative sleep stages. Factors that are associated with sleep disruption in the ICU include patient-ventilator desynchrony, medications, patient care interactions, and environmental noise and light. As the field of critical care increasingly focuses on patients' physical and psychological outcomes following critical illness, understanding the potential contribution of ICU-related sleep disruption on patient recovery is an important area of investigation.

There are many ICUs that are becoming more aware of this issue and have policies in place such as nap times, hours of the day where no visitors and limited interventions are allowed, to maximize rest. The nurse can assist in this endeavor by limiting conversations outside the patient's room if they are resting, turning off lights and closing curtains when possible, silencing alarms that are unnecessary as long as no patient risk is involved and facility policy allows, and limiting visitors when possible according to the patient's wishes.

Surveys of ICU survivors have shown that sleep deprivation and the inability to sleep rank among the top 3 major sources of anxiety and stress during the ICU stay. Studies have shown that critically ill adult patients have markedly fragmented sleep compared to healthy adults, with approximately 50% of sleep occurring during daytime hours. ICU patients commonly have broken, light sleep with a lack of restorative N3 and REM sleep.

Thermoregulation

The body maintains a healthy temperature through a process called thermoregulation. Homeostatic adjustments involved in thermoregulation include sweating to stay cool and shivering to stay warm. Healthy human temperature is somewhere near 98 degrees Fahrenheit or 37 degrees Celsius, though this may vary by a degree or so from individual to individual.

Colder than normal body temperature is called hypothermia and warmer than normal body temperature is called hyperthermia or fever. Either condition, if prolonged, may lead to death if left uncorrected. Drug and alcohol use, and hypothyroidism may lead to hypothermia, while digestion, fever, and exercise may cause hyperthermia. Exposure to extreme heat or cold in the environment can lead to hypo- or hyperthermia.

Toxin/Drug Exposure

The immune system of the body prevents disease from occurring after exposure to infectious agents. When the immune system overreacts to a substance that is not harmful, an allergic reaction occurs. Commonly occurring allergies include dust mites, insect stings, foods, plant pollen, or molds. Some patients may have allergies to types of drugs, such as penicillin and its derivatives.

An allergic reaction may include mild symptoms such as itching of the eyes, running nose, coughing, and sneezing. A more severe allergic response may include periorbital edema, wheezing, and difficulty breathing. Some allergies may be life threatening and the patient must avoid exposure to that allergen. Anaphylaxis is the term for a rare, but serious reaction to an allergen. Anaphylaxis may result in death if aggressive intervention does not take place quickly. Avoiding the allergen, if possible, will prevent allergic reactions, yet many allergens are difficult to avoid. In these cases, allergy medications may be useful. For seasonal allergies, decongestants and antihistamines are helpful in lowering the body's inflammatory response. Corticosteroids may be used to decrease inflammation in the body. For some patients, exposure therapy, where the patient is slowly, methodically exposed to their allergen in small doses. Over time it is hoped that they will develop a tolerance to the allergen and be able to handle full exposure to it after therapy is completed.

Toxic Ingestions/Inhalations

Any chemical that can cause harm to the body when ingested or inhaled is considered **toxic.** Exhaust fumes from cars, lead in drinking water, asbestos in old buildings, and pesticides on plants can all cause harm to the body if ingested or inhaled. Ingestion occurs through eating or swallowing the substance, which then travels through the body's GI tract and is absorbed into the circulatory system from the small intestine. A short-term effect would be headache and vomiting, while long-term effects could include cancer and other disease states. Substances that are inhaled travel through the airways, into the lungs, and are absorbed into the circulation through the pulmonary capillary beds.

Treatment of toxic ingestions depends on the toxic substance ingested. Stomach pumping and administration of activated charcoal may be necessary to rid the body of the toxin. Activated charcoal works by absorbing the toxin before the body gets a chance to, decreasing its toxic effects.

36/50 = 72%

Practice Questions

1. A 29-year-old female presents with severe pain in her knee joint with papules, redness, and tenderness surrounding. What type of organism does the nurse suspect has caused this acute infectious arthritis?
    a. *Neisseria gonorrhea* joint
    b. *Staphylococcus aureus* osteo
    c. *Streptococcus pyogenes* strep throat
    d. *Candida*

2. Which of the following are true regarding encephalopathy?
    I. It is complication of a primary problem.
    II. It is brain damage.
    III. It is an altered mental state.
    IV. It is caused by a lack of oxygen to the brain.

    a. Choices I, II, and III
    b. Choices I, II, and IV
    c. Choices II, III, and IV
    d. All of the above

3. Which of the following is an example of toxic substance ingestion?
    a. A child eating a Tide pod
    b. Breathing exhaust fumes
    c. Sniffing glue
    d. All of the above

4. A 35-year-old male presents with headaches, memory loss, and periods of disorientation. The nurse discovers that he played professional football for many years and is now retired. The nurse suspects which type of encephalopathy will be diagnosed?
    a. Chronic traumatic encephalopathy
    b. Hepatic encephalopathy
    c. Toxic-metabolic encephalopathy
    d. Hashimoto's encephalopathy

5. A nurse is managing the care of a patient who has been admitted for an intracranial hemorrhage. Which of the following is a likely culprit for intracranial hemorrhaging and must be carefully managed?
    a. Electrolyte imbalances
    b. Sepsis
    c. Aneurysmal rupture
    d. High blood pressure

6. Which structure of the brain is responsible for producing cerebral spinal fluid?
    a. Pons
    b. Ventricle
    c. Thalamus
    d. Corpus callosum

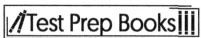

7. A patient who has experienced an ischemic stroke will likely be put on which type of drug therapy to prevent future clots from occurring?
   a. Beta blockers
   b. Statins
   c. Platelet anti-aggregants
   d. Anti-hypertensives

8. Which type of IV medication will be helpful in stabilizing the blood pressure of a patient with a subarachnoid hemorrhage?
   a. Vasopressors
   b. Beta blockers
   c. Analgesics
   d. Nitrates

9. A 25-year-old male is experiencing neck stiffness that came on rather quickly. Other symptoms include headache, malaise, and fever. The nurse suspects which type of infection is at work?
   a. Tonsillitis
   b. Laryngitis
   c. Meningitis
   d. Bronchitis

10. Which of the following is an example of a neurosurgery performed on the peripheral nervous system?
    a. Lumbar laminectomy
    b. Aneurysm clipping
    c. Conventional open surgery
    d. Carpal tunnel correction

11. Which of the following drugs is often used for treatment of acute seizure activity?
    a. Memantine HCl
    b. Phenytoin
    c. Pregabalin
    d. Rifaximin

12. Which of the following is/are true regarding vertebral osteomyelitis?
    a. It develops gradually
    b. It causes pain down the legs
    c. Pain improves with rest
    d. All of the above

13. A 9-month old baby is in the ER and shaken baby syndrome is suspected. This falls under what category of traumatic brain injury?
    a. Closed
    b. Developing
    c. Open
    d. Insidious

14. A 22-year-old male diagnosed with schizophrenia is acting out on the psych unit. He is verbally assaulting other patients, pacing nervously, and says his heart feels like it is "beating out of control!" The nurse sees that the patient is agitated and knows which intervention will be the last resort in assisting this patient?

    a. First generation antipsychotics
    b. Second generation antipsychotics
    c. Verbal de-escalation
    d. Physical restraints

15. Which of the following descriptions does NOT describe a patient diagnosed with antisocial personality disorder (ASPD)?

    a. Aggressive
    b. Reclusive
    c. Disrespectful
    d. Violent

16. Which of the following words describes delirium and differentiates it from dementia?

    a. Slow onset
    b. Irreversible
    c. Chronic
    d. Transient

17. Which psychological disorder often precedes a dementia diagnosis?

    a. Bipolar disorder
    b. Panic disorder
    c. Depressive disorder withdrawn?
    d. Schizophrenia

18. The nurse is discharging a patient with a history of medical non-adherence. He has diabetes and is known to miss follow-up appointments and lab tests to check his hemoglobin A1C. What intervention can the nurse perform to best help him adhere to his prescribed treatment plan, to better manage his diabetes?

    a. Investigate the reason for his non-adherence
    b. Quiz the patient about when his follow-up doctor appointments will be
    c. Screen the patient for a psychological diagnosis
    d. Read every page of the discharge paperwork to the patient, ensuring he listens carefully

19. A 19-year-old patient diagnosed with bipolar disorder has been admitted to the psychiatric unit following a spending spree, several counts of risky and promiscuous sex with strangers, and finally being caught shoplifting several hundred dollars' worth of clothes from a local Target. The nurse concludes that the patient was in which portion of the bipolar cycle?

    a. Anxious
    b. Depressive
    c. Mania
    d. Panic

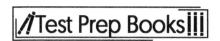

20. A 29-year-old veteran of the Marine Corps experiences a recurrent nightmare that revisits his combat experience. Last week at a 4th of July celebration in his town, he experienced a dissociative state of mind after hearing the popping of the fireworks. The nurse recognized he may have what psychological disorder?

  a. Antisocial behavior disorder
  b. Panic attack disorder
  c. Bipolar disorder
  d. Post-traumatic stress disorder

21. What did Sigmund Freud theorize was the reason behind risk-taking behavior?

  a. The desire for near-death experience
  b. Oral fixation
  c. Hysteria
  d. Repressed conflicts

22. A 49-year-old patient experiencing severe alcohol withdrawal exhibits vestibular disturbance by reporting which of the following symptoms?

  a. "I have a terrible headache."
  b. "The room is spinning!"
  c. "My hands won't stop shaking!"
  d. "I am nauseated."

23. A patient with a history of depression and suicidal ideation demonstrates a non-suicidal self-injury or NSSI by doing which of the following?

  a. Taking an entire bottle of aspirin all at one time
  b. Telling a friend that she's thought about killing herself
  c. Cutting her inner arms with a razor
  d. Ingesting copious amounts of vodka

24. A morbidly obese 25-year-old male has elected to undergo a bariatric surgery in which the stomach and duodenum will be bypassed and rerouted from a stomach pouch directly to the jejunum. Which type of bariatric procedure is this?

  a. Adjustable gastric banding
  b. Gastrectomy
  c. Liposuction
  d. Roux-en-Y gastric bypass

25. What is the most significant risk to a successful renal transplant?

  a. Family history of cancer
  b. End-stage renal disease
  c. Type A blood type
  d. Supportive caregiver

26. A patient with a terminal cancer diagnosis is placed in hospice care. Who will make his healthcare decisions when he becomes incapacitated?

  a. Hospice nurse
  b. Healthcare power of attorney
  c. Caregiver
  d. Legal guardian

27. Which type of line is used to infuse substantial amounts of medicine and fluids into the patient's bloodstream?
    a. Peripheral IV
    b. Nasogastric tube
    c. Central IV
    d. Urinary catheter

28. The best way to prevent catheter-associated urinary tract infections is to do which of the following?
    a. Measure strict intake and output while the catheter is in place
    b. Monitor the urethra for signs of infection
    c. Remove the catheter as soon as possible
    d. Follow protocol before placing the catheter

29. The critical care nurse caring for a patient on a mechanical ventilator performs all except which of the following interventions to prevent ventilator-associated pneumonia?
    a. Lays the head of the bed flat while the patient is sleeping
    b. Keeps the bed at 45-90 degrees at all times
    c. Removes the endotracheal tube as soon as the patient can tolerate breathing on their own
    d. Performs regular oral hygiene interventions

30. The nurse listens to a patient as she tells him that she feels very dizzy when she stands up and has to do so very slowly. The nurse recognizes what type of low blood pressure may be occurring?
    a. Hypovolemic
    b. Postural
    c. Neural
    d. Postprandial

31. The nurse taking care of a patient with an MRSA infection knows that multidrug-resistant organisms arise from which of the following causes?
    a. Overuse of antivirals
    b. Underuse of antivirals
    c. Underuse of antibiotics
    d. Overuse of antibiotics

32. A nurse is working in an outpatient clinic giving flu shots at the beginning of the flu season. While educating a patient on the importance of the flu vaccine, she advises that the patient get the flu vaccine administered how often?
    a. Once per lifetime
    b. Every six months
    c. Annually
    d. Every two years

33. Perioperative inoculation of bacteria into the joint describes which of the following?
    a. A post-op infection
    b. A prosthetic joint infection
    c. Infectious arthritis
    d. All of the above

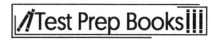

34. The critical care nurse is admitting a patient fresh out of the surgical suite following repair of multiple tears and lacerations after being stabbed several times during a gang fight. Which of the following signs signals an improvement in the patient's condition?
    a. Rise in heart rate
    b. Stabilization of blood pressure
    c. Development of fever
    d. Low urine output

35. A patient in the critical care unit tells the nurse that his pain is in his abdomen, just below the rib cage and to the right of his stomach. Which component of pain assessment has the patient reported?
    a. Location
    b. Exacerbation
    c. Alleviation
    d. Aggravation

36. A patient enters the emergency department with myalgia, stiffness, and weakness. Myoglobin is discovered in the urine and a diagnosis of rhabdomyolysis is made. The nurse would expect to see what color urine coming from the patient?
    a. Clear
    b. Light yellow
    c. Dark amber
    d. Tinged with blood

37. There is a 3% loss of muscle mass within the thigh muscles within 7 days of bedrest and contractures begin within 3 weeks. This is an example of which of the following?
    a. Immobility
    b. Decompression syndrome
    c. Deconditioning
    d. Debilitation

38. In the continuum of worsening illness, sepsis is systemic inflammatory response syndrome paired with what factor?
    a. Organ dysfunction
    b. Known source of infection
    c. Hypotensive crisis
    d. Lactic acidosis

39. What amount of blood lost is considered life threatening and will throw a patient into hypovolemic shock?
    a. 1/8
    b. 1/7
    c. 1/5
    d. 1/10

40. The patient in the ICU is having trouble sleeping due to sensory overload. The ICU nurse may do all the following interventions except:
    a. Limit visitors wherever possible
    b. Limit conversations with co-workers outside the patient's room
    c. Turn off the lights in the patient's room when they are not needed
    d. None; all of the above are appropriate interventions

41. When administering activated charcoal to a patient who has ingested a toxic substance, only give it with which of the following substances?
    a. Water
    b. Milk
    c. Sherbet
    d. Ice cream

42. Which of the following is the most likely reason for a shortened step length?
    a. Weakness of the calf muscles
    b. Weakness of the gluteal muscles
    c. Over-reliance on a walker
    d. Contractures

43. Which of the following behaviors are considered modifiable risk factors associated with increased risk of ischemic stroke?
    a. Smoking, diabetes, and cocaine use
    b. Alcoholism, sedentary lifestyle, and smoking
    c. Sedentary lifestyle, diabetes, and insulin resistance
    d. Drug use, abdominal obesity, and insulin resistance

44. Why is emergency management of subarachnoid hemorrhage so critical?
    a. Because it is caused by an aneurysm
    b. Because 10-15% of patients die before reaching the hospital
    c. Because there is bleeding between the arachnoid and dura mater layers
    d. All of the above

45. The drug Mannitol is used to treat which of the following?
    a. Cancers
    b. Status epilepticus
    c. Seizures
    d. Brain herniation

46. Which of the following is the first line of treatment for a brain tumor?
    a. Surgery
    b. Radiation therapy
    c. Chemotherapy
    d. Treatment is based on severity

47. A patient at a clinic with a BARS score of 1 requires which of the following?
    a. Verbal de-escalation techniques
    b. Further evaluation at the clinic
    c. Immediate transfer to a medical ED
    d. Environmental modification

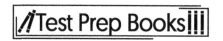

48. Goals of care conversations are used at the end of life to do which of the following?
    a. Collaborate with experts
    b. Keep the focus on what the patient wants
    c. Support families during a difficult time
    d. Get the patient into palliative care

49. Which of the following is/are true regarding advance directives?
    a. They are an expression of the patient's preferences.
    b. They based on a person's values and beliefs.
    c. They include identification of a surrogate.
    d. All of the above

50. Which of the following answers is true about pain?
    a. Pain can always be controlled by opioids
    b. Pain always causes depression
    c. Pain can slow thought processes and impair memory
    d. All of the above

Answer Explanations

1. A: *Neisseria gonorrhea* is a common cause of acute infection of a joint. *Staphylococcus aureus* is a common infectious agent in osteomyelitis. *Streptococcus pyogenes* is the causative bacterial organism in strep throat. *Candida* is the most common opportunistic invader of the fungal family.

2. A: Encephalopathy is a general term that means brain disease, damage, or malfunction, with the major symptom being an altered mental state. It is not always caused by a lack of oxygen to the brain; that is anoxic encephalopathy. However, there are other possible causes. For example, hepatic encephalopathy is caused by liver disease. Encephalopathy is often considered a complication of a primary problem.

3. A: The child ate (ingested) the toxin. Breathing fumes or sniffing glue are examples of inhalation, not ingestion.

4. A: Based on the history of playing football and the presenting symptoms, the patient likely has chronic traumatic encephalopathy or CTE. Hepatic encephalopathy results from liver dysfunction. Hashimoto's encephalopathy is a subacute condition associated with Hashimoto's thyroiditis. Toxic-metabolic encephalopathy is related to metabolic disorders and is unrelated to head trauma.

5. D: High blood pressure is the most common cause of intracranial hemorrhage, and thus is a high priority in the nurse's management of the patient. Aneurysmal rupture is a common cause in subarachnoid bleeds. Sepsis and electrolyte imbalances are unrelated to this condition.

6. A: The ventricles of the brain are responsible for the production of cerebrospinal fluid. The pons is located at the end of the brain stem and is responsible for regulating breathing. The thalamus acts as a message exchange center for the cerebrum and limbic system, and is located just above the brain stem. The corpus callosum is the fibrous tissue of white matter that connects the left and right brain.

7. C: Anti-aggregants, such as aspirin, prevent platelets from sticking together, thus preventing clotting that would lead to ischemic stroke. Anti-hypertensives and statins may be prescribed to control blood pressure and hyperlipidemia, respectively, but are not used for preventing coagulopathy. Beta blockers fall under the class of anti-hypertensives.

8. B: Beta blockers given by IV would be most appropriate in treating a patient with a subarachnoid brain hemorrhage, to stabilize blood pressure. Dopamine is a vasopressor that is used to raise blood pressure in hypotensive crises; thus, it is not appropriate in this scenario. Nitrates are often used to treat myocardial infarction to return coronary blood flow. Analgesics are used for pain control rather than controlling hypertension as this scenario presents.

9. C: Meningitis classically presents with nuchal rigidity, or neck stiffness. Laryngitis is an inflammation of the larynx and does not present with nuchal rigidity. Bronchitis, an infection of the airways, also does not cause the patient to feel stiffness of the neck. Tonsillitis, an infection of the tonsils, will have the patient feeling sore in the throat, but not stiff in the neck.

10. D: Correction of carpal tunnel syndrome would require a type of neurosurgery affecting the peripheral nervous system. Lumbar laminectomy affects the lumbar region of the spine and not the peripheral nervous system. Clipping of aneurysms usually occurs in the brain or other centralized regions

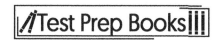

of the nervous system. Conventional open surgery involves drilling holes into the skull to access the brain tissue needing surgical intervention.

11. B: Phenytoin is the drug of choice when treating acute seizures. Memantine is a neurological drug used to treat dementia. Pregabalin is a drug used to treat diabetic neuropathy. Rifaximin is a drug used to treat hepatic encephalopathy.

12. A: Vertebral osteomyelitis develops gradually and does not improve with rest, nor does it cause pain down the legs.

13. A: Shaken baby syndrome in this case falls under the category of closed traumatic brain injury (TBI), as there is no open wound that is bleeding. A TBI that includes an open skull wound is called an open TBI. The other two terms listed do not refer to TBI and are thus not appropriate for this scenario.

14. D: The nurse will use physical restraints to calm an agitated patient as a last resort. Verbal de-escalation should be the first intervention. If the patient continues to act out aggressively and violently, antipsychotics, both first and second generation, may be used to calm the patient down. Use of restraints is a last resort intervention, and in order to do so the nurse must obtain a doctor's order and follow facility policy.

15. B: A reclusive person may have agoraphobia and social anxiety, but not antisocial personality disorder (ASPD). A person with ASPD acts out in a way that is aggressive, violent, and disrespectful toward people they are around, making them antisocial in that way.

16. D: Delirium is transient, reversible, and usually has an acute onset with an illness. Dementia, on the other hand, is a slow-developing, irreversible, and chronic condition often accompanied by another chronic diagnosis such as Parkinson's or Alzheimer's. Dementia may be slowed, but never fully reversed. Delirium usually can be treated and reversed by treating the underlying cause.

17. C: Depression is often the first sign of the development of dementia later in life. Up to forty percent of Alzheimer's patients also have a concurrent diagnosis of depression. Panic disorder, schizophrenia, and bipolar disorder may certainly occur with dementia but are not as common.

18. A: Determining the underlying cause of medical non-adherence will greatly help in promoting future adherence to the patient's treatment plan. The patient may be depressed, burnt out, socioeconomically disadvantaged, and so on. It's hard to tell without making the effort to understand him better. Reading the patient's discharge instructions out loud may do nothing to help him adhere to his medical treatment plan; in fact, he probably is already familiar with discharge instructions and would be further put off by the effort. Screening for a psychological diagnosis is inappropriate and likely outside of the nurse's scope of practice for this particular scenario. Usually facility policy or a doctor's order would be reason to perform such a screen. Quizzing the patient about discharge information is inappropriate as he may well know when his follow-up appointments are but may not have the means to make it there if his car was broken down, for example. Again, the underlying cause of the medical non-adherence needs to be discovered before any other assumptions are made.

19. C: The patient is clearly in the mania portion of the bipolar cycle, characterized by the spending spree, the promiscuous sex, and the shoplifting. The mania portion of bipolar entails a prolonged period of elation, where the patient has an inflated ego and feels that the rules no longer apply to them. Excessive behavior is characteristic of this portion of the bipolar spectrum. Depression, panic, and anxiety are different parts of the mood disorder spectrum, with different defining characteristics.

20. D: The recurrent nightmares and flashbacks that the soldier is experiencing that revisit his experiences in combat are classic symptoms of post-traumatic stress disorder, or PTSD. The soldier may experience panic attacks, but that disorder falls under a different category with different and specific symptoms. Bipolar disorder is another possibility, but again, it has its own specific symptoms that are not described in this scenario. Antisocial behavior involves acting aggressively and violently toward others, which is not the presentation described here.

21. A: Freud theorized that risk-taking behavior originates from an innate drive within humans to be near death. According to Freud, oral fixation has to do with being weaned too early and needing to do things with one's mouth such as smoking. Repressed conflicts are part of a lot of Freud's theory and thus not specific to this question. Hysteria was a broad term to describe mental illnesses of women back in Freud's time and not specific to risk-taking behavior.

22. B: All the symptoms reported by the patient are part of severe alcohol withdrawal; however, reporting that the room is spinning points towards vestibular disturbance. Patients experiencing vestibular disturbance will feel that the room is rotating, the walls are falling, and the floor is moving. The GI symptoms, headache, and tremors relate to different systems affected by the alcohol withdrawal.

23. C: Cutting her inner arms is an example of non-suicidal self-injury. NSSIs are not meant to kill oneself, but rather relieve psychological pain by inflicting physical pain on oneself. Ingesting the vodka and the aspirin are suicidal attempts, in which taking one's life is the intention. Reporting suicidal thoughts to a friend is likely a cry for help.

24. D: The procedure described is the Roux-en-Y bypass, in which the stomach is made into a smaller gastric pouch, the rest of the stomach and duodenum are completely bypassed, and the gastric pouch then empties directly into the jejunum. This procedure makes it so the patient feels fuller faster because of the smaller gastric pouch, thus decreasing caloric intake significantly and promoting weight loss. Gastrectomy, gastric banding, and liposuction are different bariatric surgeries that do not fit the description in the scenario.

25. B: The patient's concurrent end-stage renal disease is considered a comorbidity and will worsen their chances of a successful transplantation. A supportive caregiver is always good to have, but does not affect the transplant outcome significantly. Type A blood is unrelated to transplant outcomes. A family history of cancer does not affect the outcome of kidney transplantation.

26. B: Healthcare power of attorney is the legal term for the person appointed by the patient to make their healthcare decisions should they become incapacitated. This may be a caregiver, but not necessarily. The hospice nurse does not make the decisions but rather follows the doctor's orders and gives council to the patient and their family. A legal guardian may also be appointed to be the healthcare power of attorney, but not necessarily.

27. C: A central intravenous line is used to infuse substantial amounts of medicine and fluids directly into the patient's bloodstream. A peripheral IV may be used for medicine and fluids but the blood vessels located in the periphery are not large enough to handle the amount of fluids and medications the central vessels can. Nasogastric tubes may have medication placed in them, but are limited due to the medication having to travel through, and be absorbed by, the GI tract first. A urinary catheter drains urine into a bag and is used for output monitoring.

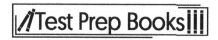

28. C: The urinary catheter must be removed as soon as possible to prevent infection from developing. Never placing the catheter in the first place would be the absolute best way to prevent infection, but that is not an option, nor is it realistic in the acute care setting. Monitoring the urethra for infection will not prevent infection. Recording intake and output does not affect infection. Following protocol before placing the catheter will help prevent careless and needless placements of catheters, but may not affect preventing infection if the catheter is not removed in a timely manner.

29. A: Laying the head of the bed flat for extended periods of time for the patient who is on mechanical ventilation is inappropriate and may put them at risk for developing ventilator-associated pneumonia, as well as possibly causing respiratory distress. The head of the bed should be elevated to 45-90 degrees at all times. Discontinuing mechanical ventilation as soon as the patient can tolerate it is ideal. Regular oral care should be performed to keep the mouth clean and prevent infections from developing.

30. B: Low blood pressure that occurs when a patient changes position from sitting to standing is called postural hypotension and may be caused by cardiac or neurological disease. Postprandial hypotension results after one eats. Neural hypotension arises from neurological deficits and is not positional. Hypovolemic hypotension is a type of low blood pressure that is caused by low circulating blood volume.

31. D: Overuse of antibiotics is what led to the mutation and uprising of drug-resistant organisms such as MRSA, VRE, and CRE. These types of "super bugs" are resistant to antibiotic treatments that used to work against them such as methicillin, amoxicillin, penicillin, and oxacillin. Stronger, broader antibiotic treatments must be used for longer periods of time to kill off drug-resistant organisms that cause infections.

32. C: The flu vaccine should be administered every year at the beginning of the flu season. Every year a strain of flu is identified as being the likely culprit for cases of the flu for that year and used in the vaccines, thus everyone six months and older should get their flu shot each and every year. The other answers are invalid.

33. B: Perioperative inoculation occurs around the time of surgery, and happens most frequently in joint replacement surgery. Although it could be considered a post op infection, its cause is perioperative and not post-operative. Infectious arthritis, a joint infection, is not exclusively the result of surgery.

34. B: Stabilization of the patient's blood pressure is an excellent sign that their condition is improving. Fever, oliguria, and tachycardia are all signs of deterioration and may point toward complications such as shock, bleeding, and/or infection, and need further investigation.

35. A: The patient has reported the location of his pain. Alleviation refers to an action that makes the pain better. Aggravation refers to an action that makes the pain worse. Exacerbation is a particularly intense flare-up of a chronic pain issue.

36. C: A patient with rhabdomyolysis will have a dark amber colored urine, resembling the color of cola. This is due to the myoglobin that leaked from the muscle tissue and was excreted in the urine. Yellow and clear colored urine are normal findings while blood-tinged urine is not a characteristic finding of rhabdomyolysis and may suggest another pathology.

37. C: Deconditioning is the term for muscle wasting and debilitation caused by bedrest. Immobility is the limited ability to move freely, which may lead to deconditioning. Decompression syndrome is a physiological condition caused by a rapid decrease in surrounding pressure and is unrelated to these symptoms. Debilitation describes a loss of strength, not necessarily muscle wasting, and thus is not the best choice to explain the described changes.

38. B: Systemic inflammatory response syndrome (SIRS) paired with a known source of infection is called sepsis. Organ dysfunction is part of severe sepsis and lactic acidosis is a hypoperfusion abnormality that presents when severe sepsis has advanced to septic shock.

39. C: Losing 1/5 or 20% percent of one's blood volume will throw a person into hypovolemic shock and is considered life threatening. Organ failure with profound hypotension will likely follow; fluid resuscitation and blood transfusions will be needed as soon as possible.

40. D: All of the choices represent ways the nurse can limit the patient's sensory input so that they can get neurologic rest.

41. A: Activated charcoal will work best if it is administered with water only. Milk, sherbet, and ice cream all have the potential to diminish its absorptive qualities, decreasing its effectiveness against the toxic substance ingested.

42. A: Weakness of the calf muscles is usually the cause of a shortened step length.

43. B: Alcoholism, sedentary lifestyle, and smoking are all risk factors that the patient can readily modify if they want to. Diabetes and insulin resistance are not things that the patient can easily change.

44. B: 10%-15% of patients who have a subarachnoid hemorrhage die before they reach the hospital. It is caused by a head injury, not an aneurysm, and bleeding occurs between the arachnoid and pia mater layers.

45. D: Mannitol is used to prevent brain herniation. It is not indicated as therapy for any of the other conditions

46. D: Treatment for a brain tumor is based upon severity of the tumor.

47. C: A patient with a BARS score of 1 is lethargic and difficult to rouse so immediate transfer to an ED is needed to determine cause.

48. B: Goals of care are held to keep the focus on what the dying patient wants at their end time.

49. D: The patient's preferences, values, and beliefs, as well as indication of a surrogate decision maker, are all included in advance directives.

50. C: Pain can slow thought processes and impair memory. It cannot always be controlled and does not always cause depression.

Professional Caring & Ethical Practice

Ethical principles are the basis for personal and professional behavior. While generally moral behavior based on ethical principles is required from all individuals in a society, nurses are held to a more stringent standard for professional practice. Professionally, nurses are responsible for applying ethical principles to the care of patients and to the support of novice nurses as they develop their own professional identity.

Advocacy/Moral Agency

The American Nurses Association (ANA) provides this definition of nursing practice: "The protection, promotion, and optimization of health and abilities, prevention of illness and injury, alleviation of suffering through the diagnosis and treatment of human response, and advocacy in the care of individuals, families, communities, and populations." The ANA also addresses the importance of advocacy in its Code of Ethics, specifically in Provision 3: "The nurse promotes, advocates for, and protects the rights, health, and safety of the patient." The ANA Code of Ethics further states: nurses must advocate "with compassion and respect for the inherent dignity, worth, and uniqueness of every individual, unrestricted by considerations of social or economic status, personal attributes, or the nature of health problems."

Advocacy is a key component of nursing practice. An **advocate** is one who pleads the cause of another; and the nurse is an advocate for patient rights. Preserving human dignity, patient equality, and freedom from suffering are the basis of nursing advocacy. Nurses are in a unique position that allows them to integrate all aspects of patient care, ensuring that concerns are addressed, standards are upheld, and positive outcomes remain the goal. An experienced nurse helps patients navigate the unfamiliar system and communicate with their physicians. Nurses educate the patient about tests and procedures and are aware of how culture and ethnicity affect the patient's experience. Nurses strictly adhere to all privacy laws.

Advocacy is the promotion of the common good, especially as it applies to at-risk populations. It involves speaking out in support of policies and decisions that affect the lives of individuals who do not otherwise have a voice. Nurses meet this standard of practice by actively participating in the politics of healthcare accessibility and delivery because they are educationally and professionally prepared to evaluate and comment on the needs of patients at the local, state, and national level. This participation requires an understanding of the legislative process, the ability to negotiate with public officials, and a willingness to provide expert testimony in support of policy decisions. The advocacy role of nurses addresses the needs of the individual patient as well as the needs of all individuals in the society, and the members of the nursing profession.

In clinical practice, nurses represent the patient's interests by active participation in the development of the plan of care and subsequent care decisions. Advocacy, in this sense, is related to patient autonomy and the patient's right to informed consent and self-determination. Nurses provide the appropriate information, assess the patient's comprehension of the implications of the care decisions, and act as the patient advocates by supporting the patient's decisions. In the critical care environment, patient advocacy requires the nurse to represent the patient's decisions even though those decisions may be opposed to those of the healthcare providers and family members.

Professionally, nurses advocate for policies that support and promote the practice of all nurses with regard to access to education, role identity, workplace conditions, and compensation. The responsibility for professional advocacy requires nurses to provide leadership in the development of the professional nursing role in all practice settings that may include acute care facilities, colleges and universities, or community agencies. Leadership roles in acute care settings involve participation in professional practice and shared governance committees, providing support for basic nursing education by facilitating clinical and preceptorship experiences, and mentoring novice graduate nurses to the professional nursing role. In the academic setting, nurses work to ensure the diversity of the student population by participating in the governance structure of the institution, conducting and publishing research that supports the positive impact of professional nursing care on patient outcomes, and serving as an advocate to individual nursing students to promote their academic success. In the community, nurses assist other nurse-providers to collaborate with government officials to meet the needs that are specific to that location.

The nurse must function as a **moral agent**. This means that the nurse must be morally accountable and responsible for personal judgment and actions. Nurses who practice with moral integrity possess a strong sense of themselves and act in ways consistent with what they understand is the right thing to do. Moral agency is defined as the ability to identify right and wrong actions based on widely accepted moral criteria. The performance of nurses as moral agents is dependent on life experiences, advanced education, and clinical experience in healthcare agencies. Moral agency involves risk. It is an action that can be at odds with the traditional role of the nurse. As nurses assume more responsibility and accountability for client management and outcomes, it is essential to approach ethical dilemmas in a manner consistent with the caring component of nursing.

The role of moral agent requires nurses to have a strong sense of self and a clear understanding of the definition of right and wrong; however, nurses must also be aware that these perceptions of right and wrong will be challenged every day. In reality, nurses who act as the moral agents and are accountable for right and wrong decisions commonly encounter situations where the correct and moral action related to the patient's right to self-determination is opposed to the right and moral action with respect to competent patient care.

Caring Practices

The introduction of nursing processes in the 1970s led to the development of nursing models in the 1990s. Generally there are three components to a nursing model: a set of core beliefs and values, a statement of the goals the nurse is trying to achieve, and the knowledge and skills the nurse needs to practice (Pearson et al, 1996). In 1995 Fawcett explained that all nursing models have four central concepts: Person (the recipient of all nursing actions); Environment (the recipient's specific surroundings); Health (wellness or illness state of the recipient); and Nursing (actions taken by nurses on behalf of or in conjunction with a recipient).

On the following page are a few of the more recent, and perhaps best known, nursing models.

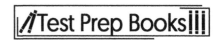

The 5 C's of Caring

The 5 C's of caring is a concept developed by Sister Simone Roach in 2002. Roach stated that nurses consistently applying the five C's in the workplace can lead to improved work relationships, improved patient relationships, and increased likelihood of career advancement.

1. Commitment: dedicated to going above and beyond normally expected behaviors; pledging to uphold the values; and commitment to pursuing life-long career learning that will enhance the level of care delivered to patients.

2. Conscience: a sense of moral responsibility resulting from a strong conscience; working consistently on another's behalf and representing the concerns of the patient; continued focus on empathy and putting yourself in the patient's shoes.

3. Competence: consistently arriving to work on time; presenting a professional manner; holding self to a high standard of excellence when fulfilling daily tasks; asking for help or clarification when there is uncertainty about a specific duty or method; continually improving skills to develop competence.

4. Compassion: empathize with patients; provide kind and considerate treatment at all times. In return, nurses may receive an inspirational sense of human connection and confirmation of the meaning of their work.

5. Confidence: confidence ties the other 4 of the 5 C's together. It takes confidence in skills and knowledge to act with commitment, follow conscience, constantly act in a competent manner, and express compassion, even in the most challenging circumstances. A confident nurse can assist others who are dealing with difficult news. A strong sense of self will summon positive change in patient care.

Family-Focused Care (Shelton and Stepanek, 1994)

1. Recognizing that the family is the constant in the patient's life while the service systems and personnel within those systems fluctuate

2. Being aware of family strengths and individuality and having respect for different methods of coping

3. Encouraging and facilitating family-to-family support and networking

4. Sharing complete and unbiased information about the patient's care with family members on a continuing basis in a supportive manner

5. Designing accessible healthcare delivery systems that are flexible, culturally competent, and responsive to family needs

The Needs of the Critical Care Family (Molter, 1997)

1. To have questions answered honestly

2. To know specific facts regarding what is wrong with the patient and their progress

3. To know the prognosis/outcome/chance of recovery

4. To be called at home about changes

5. To receive information once a day

6. To receive information and understandable explanations

7. To believe the hospital personnel care about the patient

8. To have hope

9. To know exactly what and why things are being done to the patient

10. To have reassurance that the best possible care is being given to the patient

The Synergy Model for Patient Care

The American Association of Critical-Care Nurses developed their Synergy Model for Patient Care in 1996 as a new framework for AACN's certification programs, the Synergy Model shifted the assessment of nursing skills from the then-prevalent body systems/medical model, which didn't consistently match actual practice, to a "nurse competencies" framework. The central idea of the model is that synergy results when the needs and characteristics of a patient, clinical unit or system are matched with a nurse's competencies. A patient's needs drive the nurse competencies required for patient care.

AACN Synergy Model

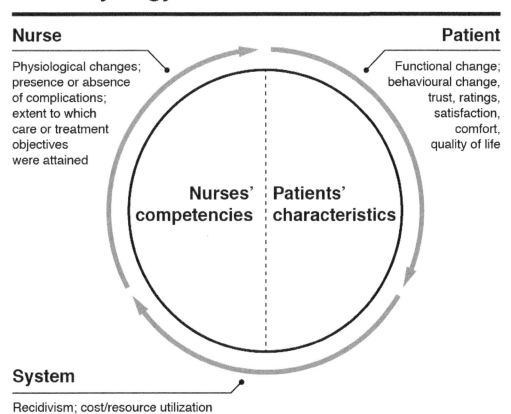

Nurse

Physiological changes; presence or absence of complications; extent to which care or treatment objectives were attained

Patient

Functional change; behavioural change, trust, ratings, satisfaction, comfort, quality of life

Nurses' competencies : Patients' characteristics

System

Recidivism; cost/resource utilization

There are five assumptions that guide the AACN Synergy Model of Nursing:

1. Patients are biological, psychological, social, and spiritual entities who present at a particular developmental stage. The whole patient must be considered.

2. The patient, family, and community all contribute to providing a context for the nurse-patient relationship.

3. Patients can be described by a number of characteristics, and all characteristics are connected and contribute to each other. Characteristics cannot be looked at in isolation.

4. Nurses can be described on a number of dimensions, and the interrelated dimensions create a profile of the nurse.

5. A goal of nursing is to restore a patient to an optimal level of wellness as defined by the patient. Death can be an acceptable outcome, in which the goal of nursing is to move the patient toward a peaceful death.

The Synergy Model also identifies the following 8 patient characteristics and 8 nurse competencies. Each of these can be evaluated on a continuum of 1-5.

The American Hospital Association's Patient Care Partnership Document

Although not a nursing care model, The American Hospital Association's Patient Care Partnership Document produced in 2005 mandated a decision-making partnership between the healthcare system and the patient, facilitating patients' efforts to determine their own future. This decision-making partnership highlighted the responsibilities of the healthcare system to fully communicate treatment options and the plan of care and mandated a change in care patterns and nursing practices.

The model identifies vigilance and engagement as essential elements. Vigilance as a caring skill is viewed on a continuum according to the ability of nurses to recognize and respond to patient needs. Novice nurses are capable of responding to usual and predictable changes in the patient's condition; however, responding to more subtle cues requires an increased level of clinical competence, and preventing any

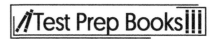

potential hazards requires even greater nursing skill. Engagement in the nurse-patient relationship refers to the degree to which nurses commit to the relationship. Researchers note that favorable patient outcomes are associated with the degree of caregiver engagement; however, there is also evidence that the incidence of burnout in experienced nurses is related to the degree of their engagement in patient care. The third attribute of the caring practices is responsiveness, which means that the reaction of the patient's family, the healthcare institution, and the nursing staff will all have an effect on the patient's progress.

Response to Diversity

National League for Nursing believes that diversity and quality health care are inseparable and together they create a path to increased access, improved health, and elimination of health disparities. Diversity signifies that each individual is unique and recognizes individual differences such as race, ethnicity, gender, sexual orientation, gender identity, socio-economic status, age, physical abilities, and religious and/or political beliefs. The result is self-awareness and respect for all persons, embracing and celebrating the richness of each individual. It also encompasses organizational, institutional, and system-wide behaviors in nursing, nursing education, and health care.

The Agency for Healthcare Research and Quality (AHRQ) states that health care quality remains suboptimal for diverse populations in the United States because some individuals do not receive quality care or believe that their values are honored or respected. The Patient Protection and Affordable Care Act (ACA) of 2010 expanded coverage and improved access to the nation's health care system. ACA's creation of subsidies made insurance more affordable and benefited immigrant citizens. The sheer numbers of immigrants coming into the health care system create enormous opportunities to provide culturally competent care.

Culture can be defined as learned and shared beliefs, values, and life ways of a designated or particular group that are generally transmitted inter-generationally and influence one's thinking and action modes. Culture can be the lens that the person uses to view the world, including health and the need for care. Cultural competence of the healthcare workforce and the healthcare delivery system is increasingly tied to improved client outcomes and quality of care provided. Cultural competence is the ability to provide effective care for patients who come from different cultures. It requires sensitivity and effective communication in both verbal and non-verbal communication. Financial reimbursement for care provided to clients can be negatively affected if there is not a system in place to support the culturally competent delivery of care.

A culturally-competent clinical nurse will develop an awareness of, and sensitivity to, their own cultural heritage and recognize how their own values and biases may affect patients. The nurse is expected to do the following:

- Demonstrate comfort with cultural differences
- Know specifics about the cultural groups they work with
- Respect and be aware of the unique needs of specific women, men and children
- Understand that diversity exists within and between cultures
- Try to understand other points of view
- Demonstrate flexibility and tolerance, be nonjudgmental
- Maintain a sense of humor

- Demonstrate a willingness to relinquish control
- Promote cultural practices that are potentially helpful

Nurses are aware that unmet cultural or diversity needs and preferences can adversely affect patient outcomes in much the same way that somatic illness affects outcomes. Therefore, cultural sensitivity is an essential nurse competency. The development of cultural sensitivity and demonstrated appreciation of diversity by nurses is also viewed as a continuum in the Synergy Model. Novice nurses, who are learning to negotiate the institutional environment, may assess the patient's preferences but often continue to provide care that is consistent with their own belief system. As competent nurses gain life and clinical experience, they actively question patients to learn about and accommodate the traditions and customs of a diverse population, while helping the patient and family to understand the culture of the institution. Expert nurses are able to anticipate the needs of the patient and family by integrating cultural differences into the plan of care whenever possible. All of these nursing interventions work to alleviate the stress related to the acute care environment.

Research indicates that diversity in the workplace strengthens the workgroup by allowing consideration of multiple worldviews and a better understanding of the patient population served by the institution. Multiple viewpoints can also be an advantage in conflict resolution, especially when the conflict is related to diversity issues. The Synergy Model suggests that nurses become more sensitive to diversity issues with experience and that this sensitivity is applicable to the work environment as well as direct patient care. Attention to diversity issues also, however, requires institutional support for resource allocation and management. Depending on the specific needs of the patient population, services such as foreign language interpreters, appropriate food service, counseling services, and accommodation for religious observances must be considered. To optimize patient care, expert nurses assess the needs of the patient and family, and provide access to the appropriate institutional resources.

Attention to diversity issues requires that providers proceed on the assumption that ethnocentrism is a universal human characteristic that must be addressed by the provision of appropriate information and instruction. In addition to understanding their own cultural views, nurses must be aware that many patients have preconceived views of western cultural norms, which may or may not be accurate, but can potentially affect the nurse-patient relationship. The resolution of ethnocentrism in a caring relationship requires acknowledgment of its existence and education as to the meaning of the traditions and practices.

Facilitation of Learning

Facilitation of learning refers to the process of assessing the learning needs of the patient and family, the nursing staff, and caregivers in the community, and creating, implementing, and evaluating formal and informal educational programs to address those needs. Novice nurses often view patient care and patient education as separate entities; however, experienced nurses are able to integrate the patient's educational needs into the plan of care. Nurses are aware that the patient often requires continued reinforcement of the educational plan after discharge, which necessitates coordination with home care services.

As facilitators of learning, nurses may be involved in a large-scale effort to educate all patients over 65 admitted to the nursing unit about the need for both Prevnar 13 and Pneumovax 23 to prevent pneumonia. In contrast, nurses may provide one-on-one instruction for a patient recently diagnosed with diabetes. The first step of any teaching-learning initiative is the assessment of the learning needs of the participants. Specific needs that influence the design and content of the educational offering include the language preference and reading level of the participants. Nurses must also consider the effect of certain patient characteristics identified in the Synergy Model on the patient's capacity to process information. Diminished resiliency or stability, and extreme complexity, must be considered in the development of the educational plan. Nurses are also responsible for creating a bridge between teaching-learning in the acute care setting and the home environment. A detailed discharge plan, close coordination with outpatient providers, and follow-up phone calls to the patient may be used to reinforce the patient's knowledge of the plan of care.

Successful learning plans for staff members and colleagues also consider the motivation of the participants to engage in the process. Successful facilitators include a variety of teaching strategies to develop the content and evaluate learning, in order to address adult learning needs and preferences, such as preferred language and reading level. Research indicates that when adults do not have a vested interest in the outcomes of the teaching/learning process, they may not participate as active learners.

The remaining element of successful facilitation of learning is the availability and quality of learning resources. There is evidence that individuals with different learning styles respond differently to various learning devices. The minimum requirements for successful facilitation of learning include the skilled staff to develop the educational materials, paper, a copy machine, and staff to interact with the patient in the learning session.

Barriers to the facilitation of learning must be anticipated and accommodated. Changes in the patient's condition commonly require reduction in the time spent in each learning session due to fatigue. Cognitive impairment can impede comprehension and retention of the information and will require appropriate teaching aids. The learning abilities of the patient's family members must also be assessed. Adequate instruction time might be the greatest barrier. Learning needs are assessed and discharge planning is begun on the day of admission; however, shortened inpatient stays require evaluation of the patient's comprehension of the plan of care.

Collaboration

The integration of physical and mental health care is an important aspect of the Medical Home, also known as the Medicaid health home model. The model shows collaborative care programs as an approach to integration in which primary care providers, care managers, and psychiatric consultants work together to provide care and monitor patient progress. These programs have been shown to be both clinically-effective and cost-effective for a variety of mental health conditions, in a variety of settings, using several different payment mechanisms.

Some of the benefits of collaboration include improved patient outcomes, decreased healthcare costs, decreased length of stay, improved patient and nurse satisfaction, and improved teamwork. Collaboration related to patient care has been widely studied and is considered as both a process and an outcome, which occurs when no single individual is able to solve a patient problem. Collaboration as a process is defined as a synthesis of diverse opinions and skills that is employed to solve complex problems. As an outcome, collaboration is defined as a complex solution to a problem that requires the expertise of more than one individual. This view of collaboration characterizes the process as a series of actions by more than one individual, which creates a solution to a complex problem.

Initially, all members of the collaborative team must identify their own biases and acknowledge the effect of these mental models on the decision-making process. In addition, members must also be aware that the complexity of the problem will be matched by the complexity of the mental models of the collaborative team members, which will influence the decision-making process. It is also essential for team members to recognize the elements of diversity in the group. For instance, while stereotyping is obviously to be avoided, there are gender differences that should be considered. Research indicates that men tend to be more task oriented, and women tend to be more relationship oriented in the problem-solving process; this means that consideration of both points of view is necessary for genuine collaboration. Another requisite skill of the collaborative team is the development and usage of conflict resolution skills, which are required to counteract this common barrier to effective collaboration. Team members are required to separate the task from the emotions in the discussion. Effective collaboration also requires that members of the team display a cooperative effort that works to create a win/win situation, while recognizing that collaboration is a series of activities that require time and patience for satisfactory completion.

Common barriers to effective collaboration include conflicting professional opinions, ineffective communication related to the conflict, and incomplete assessment of the required elements of the care plan. Research indicates that physicians tend to stress cure-related activities while nurses tend to encourage care-related activities. This means that some resolution of these differences is required for effective communication. Although the Synergy Model defines collaboration as a necessary part of the process that matches the patient needs with the appropriate nursing competencies, it is also possible that the end product may be the best solution for the patient and at the same time be totally unacceptable to the patient. Collaborative team members should also be aware that while successful collaboration improves patient outcomes, research indicates that genuine collaborative efforts are rarely noted in patient care, often because the group is unable to integrate the diverse mental models of the group members.

Systems Thinking

The Iceberg

A Tool for Guiding Systematic Thinking

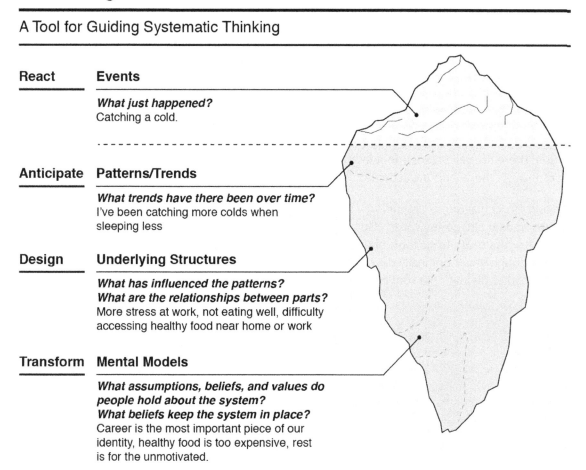

React	**Events**	
	What just happened?	
	Catching a cold.	
Anticipate	**Patterns/Trends**	
	What trends have there been over time?	
	I've been catching more colds when sleeping less	
Design	**Underlying Structures**	
	What has influenced the patterns?	
	What are the relationships between parts?	
	More stress at work, not eating well, difficulty accessing healthy food near home or work	
Transform	**Mental Models**	
	What assumptions, beliefs, and values do people hold about the system?	
	What beliefs keep the system in place?	
	Career is the most important piece of our identity, healthy food is too expensive, rest is for the unmotivated.	

Systems thinking is defined as a link between individuals and their environment. For nurses, this refers to their ability to understand the influence of the healthcare environment on patient outcomes. Systems thinking is identified as the goal of all of the Quality and Safety Education for Nurses (QESN) competencies, which are acquired by nurses on a continuum that ranges from the care of the individual patient to the care of the entire patient population. The QESN competencies were originally identified to improve patient outcomes in response to extensive research that identified a significant difference between the care of patients and the improvement in patient outcomes resulting from that care. The nursing competencies include patient-centered care, evidence-based practice, teamwork and collaboration, safety, quality and improvement, and informatics. Successful interventions associated with each of these criteria for professional nursing practice require the ability to apply the systems thinking approach to care.

Competency related to systems thinking requires appropriate education and clinical experience, and is also identified as one of the nursing competencies in the Synergy Model. In that model, novice nurses view the patient and family as isolated in the nursing unit rather than being influenced by the healthcare system, while experienced nurses are able to integrate all of the resources in the healthcare system to improve patient outcomes. Several of the learning activities designed to improve nurses' ability to acquire systems thinking include creation of a grid that identifies the nursing competencies across the continuum from isolated, individual care to the level of care associated with systems thinking. There are assessment models that apply this exercise to specialty care units such as emergency care, long-term care, and outpatient care, which identify specific systems needs for these areas. Other exercises include tracking unit statistics for the QESN competencies followed by the creation, implementation, and evaluation of a plan that applies systems thinking to address that competency. All of these activities help nurses integrate patient needs with all available resources in order to improve outcomes.

Root cause analysis can also be used as a learning exercise for systems theory because this process, which is commonly used to investigate errors, looks at all elements of an institution's relationship with the error. Case studies and reflection are also recommended as useful learning aids for systems thinking. In addition, there are valid assessment instruments that can be used to assess systems thinking skills acquired through these learning activities.

A cause and effect diagram examines why something happened or might happen by organizing potential causes into smaller categories. It can also be useful for showing relationships between contributing factors. One of the seven basic tools of quality, it is referred to as a fishbone diagram or Ishikawa diagram. Although it was originally developed as a quality control tool, in the healthcare setting the diagram is used to discover the root cause of a problem, uncover bottlenecks in a process or identify where and why a process isn't working. This is called a **root cause analysis** or a **cause and effect analysis**.

Example of a Root Cause Analysis

Environment

High noise level

Location of medication room

Communication

Transcription error

Handwritten order illegible

Equipment

Medication dispensing not automated

People

Medication nurse working overtime

Leadership

Equipment needs not met

Budget constraints

Procedures

Pharmacist review not done before dispensing

Order entry not computerized

Medication Error

The root cause analysis (RCA) is used when there is an adverse event, a sentinel event, or close call in the medical setting. It can also be used when there is a concern about a process due to repeated errors, when there is a possibility of serious errors and when there are high cost errors. The RCA answers the following critical questions:

- What happened or is still happening?
- How did it happen?
- Why did it happen?
- How can we prevent it from happening again?
- What can we learn from this?

Clinical Inquiry

Clinical inquiry is an ongoing process that evaluates and challenges clinical practice in order to propose the needed change. Clinical inquiry has several components or attributes, including critical thinking, clinical reasoning, clinical judgment, critical reasoning and judgment, and creative thinking. The process is viewed as the critical structure for the establishment of evidenced based practice and quality improvement efforts. In the Synergy Model, professional nurses employ clinical inquiry to innovate and facilitate interventions that are appropriate to patient care needs. Clinical inquiry is a rigorous process that requires attention to the rules of nursing research, such as attention to sample size, and a correct match among the data, the study design, and the statistical measures. When used to implement evidenced based practice, clinical inquiry can result in replacing an outdated, even counter-productive nursing intervention with an intervention that effectively addresses the needs of the patient. Nurses who are involved in this form of clinical inquiry are viewed as evaluators and innovators in the Synergy Model. Matching patient needs with nursing competencies means that professional nurses are responsible for challenging all nursing interventions to be sure that they represent current best practice standards. As innovators, nurses are in the best position to research, implement, and evaluate alternative care practices.

Nurses acquire clinical inquiry skills on a continuum that is based on education and clinical experience. As is the case with the other nursing competencies included in the Synergy Model, this progressive development is consistent with Benner's novice to expert model that views the development of nursing expertise as a progressive process that requires ongoing education and clinical experience. Novice nurses are able to implement clinical innovations developed by others, to identify their own learning needs, and to enlist the aid of other nurses to identify critical needs of the patient. Experienced nurses are able to question the adequacy of interventions and to begin to challenge the "we have always done it this way" philosophy that is the most common rationale for many nursing interventions. They are also able to assess the utility of alternative interventions. The Synergy Model views the practice of expert nurses as the point at which clinical inquiry and clinical reasoning become inseparable elements of clinical practice. Expert nurses are able to predict changes in the patient's condition that require revision the plan of care, and are also able to develop and implement alternative approaches to address those changes.

Public funds are the most common source of research funding, which means that researchers are obligated to design studies that provide valid results that are applicable to some form of patient care and to disseminate the results appropriately. Common barriers to nursing research efforts include inadequate funding, limited access to appropriate patient populations, and lack of institutional support for research initiatives. The rapid expansion of new knowledge from multiple sources can also inhibit the assimilation and application of new care interventions by expert nurses. In addition, the final step of the clinical inquiry process, knowledge translation or dissemination, may be the most important step. Knowledge translation refers to the complex process of synthesizing the research findings, disseminating those findings to others, and integrating the findings into clinical practice. Barriers to this process include lack of rigor in the original research design with respect to sample size, data interpretation, and the applicability of the research findings. The failure of nursing researchers to access all possible modes of the dissemination of study results has also been identified as a significant barrier to the application of new interventions. All of these system-wide and individual barriers potentially limit the use of innovative patient care interventions.

Practice Questions

1. CCRN practice is based on the principles of ethical behavior. Which of the following correctly identifies the moral principle that may require knowledge of the legislative process?
    a. Fidelity
    b. Autonomy
    c. Advocacy
    d. Beneficence

2. Nurses are responsible for which of the following elements of informed consent?
    a. Identification of alternatives to the planned procedure
    b. Description of associated risks and benefits
    c. Explanation of the planned procedure or diagnostic test
    d. Assessment of the patient's understanding of the information that is provided

3. Which of the following correctly identifies a critical distinction between the two concepts of advocacy and moral agency?
    a. Advocacy is legally binding.
    b. Moral agency requires accountability for right and wrong decisions.
    c. Advocacy is implied in the paternalistic view of patient care.
    d. Moral agency only refers to support for at-risk populations.

4. Which of the following ethical principles is MOST closely related to advocacy?
    a. Distributive justice
    b. Beneficence
    c. Nonmaleficence
    d. Fidelity

5. Which of the following word pairs identifies the C's of caring practices that are most closely associated with the critical care certification in nursing?
    a. Compassion and curiosity
    b. Confidence and collaboration
    c. Conscience and creativity
    d. Commitment and competence

6. The Synergy Model views the practice of expert nurses as which of the following?
    a. Being able to anticipate the patient needs
    b. Being able to address change
    c. The point where clinical reasoning and clinical inquiry are inseparable
    d. Being able to incorporate research findings

7. When used to implement evidenced-based practice, clinical inquiry can result in which of the following?
    a. Replacing an outdated nursing intervention
    b. The nurse becoming an innovator
    c. Matching patient needs with nursing competencies
    d. All the above

8. A nurse is caring for a patient who had a colectomy two days ago. While assisting the patient back to bed, the nurse notes that the patient's heart rate and respiratory rate are slightly elevated, and the patient states, "I can feel my pulse." The nurse assesses the patient for additional signs of heart failure. This intervention is an example of which of the following caring practices according to the Synergy Model?

    a. Engagement by a novice nurse

    b. Vigilance by an experienced nurse

    c. An expected response to predictable changes by the novice nurse

    d. Collaboration by an experienced nurse

9. When is root cause analysis used?

    a. When anything goes wrong in the medical setting

    b. When there are adverse events or close calls

    c. When the doctor orders one

    d. Only when a patient death or serious injury occurs

10. How might an institution best support diversity?

    a. By requiring all employees to speak a second language

    b. By providing mandatory cultural sensitivity training for all managers

    c. By offering alternative food services

    d. By providing alternative solutions to all patient requests

11. A novice nurse is caring for a patient who requires a blood transfusion. The patient, however, has refused the transfusion due to a religious objection to the therapy. The nurse says, "I don't understand why the patient's sister can't donate the blood. No one should object to receiving blood from a family member when you need it." Which of the following statements correctly identifies the critical issue in this situation?

    a. The nurse is displaying an ethnocentric attitude.

    b. The nurse thinks that the patient is concerned about contracting an infectious disease.

    c. The nurse thinks that the patient doesn't understand the necessity of the blood transfusion.

    d. The nurse believes that blood donation from family members is safe.

12. What are the four steps of systems thinking in order?

    a. Anticipate, design, transform, react

    b. React, anticipate, design, transform

    c. Design, anticipate, react, transform

    d. Transform, react, anticipate, design

13. According to the Synergy Model, which of the following choices is associated with the patient's vulnerability?

    a. The patient is financially stable.

    b. The patient smoked cigarettes for thirty years prior to quitting five years ago.

    c. The patient is married.

    d. The patient actively participates in decisions related to the plan of care.

14. A nurse is developing a plan of care for a patient population that is culturally diverse. Which statement correctly identifies the appropriate nursing actions?
    a. The nurse follows the standard protocol for the predominant culture of the community.
    b. The nurse focuses on the cultural needs of the largest group in the population.
    c. The nurse Identifies and acknowledges self-biases and addresses the needs of the patient.
    d. The nurse meets the needs of the group according to personal values and beliefs.

15. Which of the following statements is consistent with the Synergy Model?
    a. Family participation in patient care improves outcomes.
    b. The model is based on the condition of patients and the function of the nursing staff.
    c. The model only relates to critical care environments.
    d. Synergy exists when the environment and nursing competencies are consistent with the needs of the patient and the patient's family.

16. Common barriers to effective collaboration include which of the following?
    a. Incomplete care
    b. Cure vs care activities
    c. Conflicting professional opinions
    d. All the above

17. Why did the AACN develop their Synergy Model?
    a. To match nursing practice to competencies
    b. To shift from the care model
    c. To standardize accreditation
    d. All the above

18. Which of the following statements is consistent with the QESN competencies?
    a. Using systems thinking increases collaboration.
    b. Systems thinking is the goal of all nursing competencies.
    c. Successful application of all QESN nursing competencies will improve patient safety.
    d. The ability to use systems thinking is dictated by the nurse's level of basic nursing education.

19. Which of the following potentially provides the most comprehensive view of the institution?
    a. Root cause analysis
    b. Competency grids
    c. Process diagrams
    d. Case studies

20. The American Hospital Association's Patient Care Partnership mandates which of the following?
    a. How hospitals communicate with families
    b. Responsibility for caring for terminal patients
    c. A decision-making partnership between patients and healthcare system
    d. Access to affordable insurance for everyone

21. Which of the following statements is consistent with clinical inquiry in the Synergy Model?
    a. Novice nurses begin to compare and contrast alternative solutions to patient problems.
    b. Changes in clinical practice result from clinical experience and applying research findings.
    c. Clinical inquiry is critical to the care of the vulnerable patient.
    d. The model identifies clinical inquiry as identical to clinical reasoning.

22. "The protection, promotion, and optimization of health and abilities, prevention of illness and injury, alleviation of suffering through the diagnosis and treatment of human response, and advocacy in the care of individuals, families, communities, and populations." This statement is best described as which of the following?
    a. The ANA Code of Ethics
    b. The AACN definition of clinical care
    c. The ANA definition of nursing practice
    d. The five assumptions of the Synergy Model

23. Which of the following nursing interventions is most consistent with the competencies of caring practices, advocacy, and moral agency?
    a. Developing cultural awareness of care team members
    b. Mentoring novice nurses in the use of research findings
    c. Facilitating the patient's transition from one level of care to another on the health continuum
    d. Refining educational programs for patients and families

24. According to the Synergy Model, at what level of nursing competence do the nursing competencies of clinical inquiry and clinical reasoning become inseparable in the research process?
    a. The experienced nurse
    b. The novice nurse
    c. The expert nurse
    d. The two competencies are linked in all levels of competency.

25. Which of the following has NOT been identified as a barrier to the application of nursing research findings to clinical practice?
    a. Inadequate funding
    b. Insufficient translation
    c. Lack of qualified nursing staff
    d. Limited patient populations

26. Which of the following is cited as the MOST common source of funding for nursing research?
    a. Pharmaceutical companies
    b. Public funds
    c. Non-profit organizations
    d. Private institutions

27. Which of the following is/are true regarding the Medical Home model?
    a. It is the model Medicaid uses.
    b. It incorporates collaborative care.
    c. It has been proven cost-effective in mental health care.
    d. All of the above

28. Which of the following statements is consistent with the concept of moral agency?
    a. The patient's decisions will always be honored.
    b. Nurses assume accountability for their decisions.
    c. Institutions rarely act as moral agents.
    d. Advocacy and moral agency are interchangeable concepts.

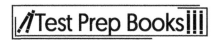

29. Research indicates which of the following regarding diversity in the workplace?
    a. It requires more money
    b. It encourages competition
    c. It strengthens the workgroup
    d. It must be led by management

30. Which of the following choices is most consistent with nurses' responsibilities for advocacy?
    a. Notify the nursing supervisor of any conflict to assure resolution of the patient issue.
    b. Consider the patient's point of view and support and explain the point of view as needed.
    c. Provide comprehensive documentation of the patient's care in the EHR.
    d. Understand all relevant laws associated with the nursing care of the patient.

Answers Explanations

1. C: Advocacy involves supporting appropriate programs and actions for marginalized or at-risk populations. At the community level, the role of advocate for the CCRN may require knowledge of the legislative process to bring about change. In direct patient care, the CCRN will be the advocate for the patient by providing the information necessary for informed choices and supporting those choices in the development of the plan of care. Fidelity refers to trust. Autonomy refers to the right of self-determination. Beneficence refers to acting in the best interest of other individuals in society.

2. D: While the physician is legally responsible for satisfying all elements of informed consent, nurses are ethically responsible for assessing the patient's ability to process and understand the implications of informed consent. Nurses protect the patient's autonomy by raising these questions and concerns. The remaining elements of informed consent are required of the physician, rather than the nurses.

3. B: Moral agency refers to decision-making that includes accountability for right and wrong decisions by the moral agent. Advocacy is an ethical principle that is not legally enforced. However, many argue that paternalism is contrary to advocacy because of the assumption that the "system" knows what is best for the patient without concern for the patient's wishes. Moral agency is not restricted to a specific population; however, the CCRN will assess the ability of all patients to make informed decisions.

4. A: Distributive justice refers to the allocation of scarce resources and advocacy is support for policies that protect at-risk populations. The CCRN understands that scarce resource allocation may be sub-standard in certain populations. In nursing, nonmaleficence means non-harming or inflicting the least harm possible to reach a beneficial outcome. Fidelity refers to faithfulness, but does not specifically address resources or the patient population.

5. D: The CCRN demonstrates professional competence as a result of a commitment to lifelong learning that is required for expert critical care nursing. The other choices each contain only a single element of the five elements of caring: commitment, conscience, competence, compassion, and confidence.

6. C: Expert nurses are those who reach the point in their clinical practice where clinical reasoning and inquiry are intertwined, allowing the nurse to make clinical judgements quickly and appropriately, according to best practice standards.

7. D: When used to implement evidenced based practice, clinical inquiry can result in replacing an outdated, even counter-productive nursing intervention with an intervention that effectively addresses the needs of the patient. Matching patient needs with nursing competencies means that professional nurses are responsible for challenging all nursing interventions to be sure that they represent current best practice standards. As innovators, nurses are in the best position to research, implement, and evaluate alternative care practices.

8. B: Vigilance refers to the ability of the nurse to recognize and respond to changes in the patient's condition. According to the Synergy Model, vigilance as a caring practice is a learned behavior that evolves with clinical experience, which means that the novice nurse will identify predictable alterations in the patient's condition, while the experienced nurse will identify and respond to more subtle changes. The most experienced nurse is capable of intervening to prevent some adverse events. Engagement refers to committing to the patient care relationship, rather than responding to changes in the patient's condition. The changes noted in the patient's condition are early, subtle indications of heart failure. The novice nurse would initially associate the changes with the surgical procedure, while the experienced nurse would assess the patient for heart failure. Although collaboration with other providers may have been an outcome of the nurse's assessment, the initial care was an independent action.

9. B: The root cause analysis is used when there is an adverse event, a sentinel event, or close call in the medical setting. It can also be used when there is a concern about a process due to repeated errors, when there is a possibility of serious errors and when there are high cost errors.

10. C: The institution can support diversity by providing resources that satisfy cultural practices such as dietary rules. Institutions also may provide interpreters, information sessions for employees, and accommodations for religious observances. Under normal circumstances, requiring employees to speak a second language would severely limit the pool of eligible employees and would not be an effective strategy. Educational programs should be provided for all employees and should not be limited to supervisory staff. Offering alternative solutions to all requests for accommodation could be viewed as paternalistic and culturally insensitive. The institution is required to consider ways to satisfy all reasonable patient requests.

11. A: The novice nurse is comparing their own beliefs to the patient's beliefs and lacks the knowledge to understand the patient's point of view. This is the definition of ethnocentrism, which can adversely affect the nurse-patient relationship. The remaining observations could potentially affect the patient's refusal of the therapy; however, the patient's refusal in this example is clearly related to the religious objection.

12. B: The four steps in systems thinking in order are react (to events); anticipate (patterns, trends, causes); design (identify the underlying structures and patterns of influence); and transform (change the beliefs and mental models).

13. B: According to the systems thinking model, vulnerability refers to the presence of any stressor, actual or potential, that could adversely affect the patient's health. A history of smoking increases the patient's vulnerability to additional health alterations. Socioeconomic status and being married are related to resource availability, which refers to the availability of financial and emotional resources that are necessary to support the patient's recovery. The patient's active participation in the plan of care is considered to have a positive effect on care outcomes.

14. C: Nurses must acknowledge their own biases and recognize that those biases will affect their ability to provide culturally sensitive care. Standard protocols related to cultural beliefs and practices are an imperfect solution to the problem of culturally sensitive care because they are not individualized to the specific patient. Meeting the needs of the largest group in a population generally means that the cultural needs of the minority groups within the population are not met. As previously stated, culturally competent care results when caregivers first consider their own biases and the possible effect of those beliefs on patient care. If nurses base their care only on their own beliefs, the patient's beliefs and practices will be ignored.

15. D: The major premise of the Synergy Model states that synergy—optimum health—can only be achieved when agency resources and nursing competencies are congruent with the patient's needs.

16. D: Common barriers to effective collaboration include conflicting professional opinions, ineffective communication related to the conflict, and incomplete assessment of the required elements of the care plan. Research indicates that physicians tend to stress "cure" related activities while nurses tend to encourage "care" related activities, which means that some resolution of these differences is required for effective communication.

17. A: The central idea of the model is that synergy results when the needs and characteristics of a patient, clinical unit or system are matched with a nurse's competencies. A patient's needs drive the nurse competencies required for patient care.

18. C: The QESN competencies were originally identified to improve patient safety in response to research that indicated that nearly 100,000 people died each year as a result of provider errors. The QESN competencies refer to nursing activities and are often used as the basis for undergraduate nursing curricula. Systems thinking is the process by which nurses meet the competencies, and attainment of this ability is an incremental process based on nurses' continuing education and clinical experiences. Although systems thinking is associated with the QESN competencies, and the use of systems thinking has improved patient outcomes, the basic assumption of the QESN competencies was improved patient safety as a result of expert nursing care.

19. A: Root cause is a structured examination of an incident or procedure that is focused on identifying the point at which an error occurred. The process is based on a comprehensive review of all parts of the organizational structure, which would support nurses understanding of the systems thinking. Competency grids, process diagrams, and case studies are strategies that measure nursing competence related to the QESN patient safety criteria.

20. C: The American Hospital Association's Patient Care Partnership document mandated a decision-making partnership between the healthcare system and the patient, facilitating patients' efforts to determine their own future. This decision-making partnership highlighted the responsibilities of the healthcare system to fully communicate treatment options and the plan of care and mandated a change in care patterns and nursing practices.

21. B: The Synergy model identifies clinical inquiry as a nursing competency that develops as a result of clinical experience and enables nurses to apply research findings to clinical practice. Novice nurses in the model are able to identify changes in the patient's condition, but do not have the skill to identify alternative interventions. Nursing competencies that are identified as critical to the care of vulnerable patients include advocacy, moral agency, collaboration, and systems thinking. Clinical reasoning is not discussed in the Synergy Model; however, clinical judgment is identified as an essential element of the clinical inquiry competency of expert nurses.

22. C: The statement provided in the question is ANA definition of nursing practice: "The protection, promotion, and optimization of health and abilities, prevention of illness and injury, alleviation of suffering through the diagnosis and treatment of human response, and advocacy in the care of individuals, families, communities, and populations."

23. C: Facilitating a patient's transition from one point on the health continuum to another requires caring practices in addition to advocacy and moral agency. Moral agency may be employed to ensure that the patient's wishes are considered, especially those wishes associated with end-of-life concerns. Developing cultural awareness is an example of a response to diversity, and the remaining two choices refer to the facilitation of learning.

24. C: The Synergy Model identifies expert nursing practice as the level of nursing competency in which clinical reasoning becomes an integrated element in the process of clinical inquiry. According to the model, prior to that point, nurses are capable of performing at some level of clinical inquiry and may be able to use clinical reasoning in patient care, but the total integration of the two does not occur until the expert level of nursing practice.

25. B: Insufficient translation is not a common barrier to the application of nursing research in clinical practice. Common barriers include inadequate funding, limited access to appropriate patient populations, lack of institutional support for research initiatives, and the rapid expansion of new knowledge from multiple sources.

26. B: Research indicates that public funds are the most common source of funding, which means that researchers are obligated to design studies that provide valid results that are applicable to some form of patient care and to disseminate the results appropriately. The remaining sources also provide funding, however public funds are noted to be the most common source.

27. D: The integration of physical and mental health care is an important aspect of the Medical Home, also known as the Medicaid health home model. The model shows collaborative care programs as an approach to integration in which primary care providers, care managers, and psychiatric consultants work together to provide care and monitor patient progress. These programs have been shown to be both clinically-effective and cost-effective for a variety of mental health conditions, in a variety of settings, using several different payment mechanisms.

28. B: When nurses act as moral agents they are required to also assume responsibility for their decisions. The patient's opinions will be identified and accommodated whenever possible; however, there may be conflict between the patient's opinions and the recommended plan of care. The institution may act as the moral agent for patients without any social support. The difference between moral agency and advocacy is the element of accountability. Moral agents are required to take responsibility for their decisions.

29. C: Research indicates that diversity in the workplace strengthens the workgroup by allowing consideration of multiple worldviews and a better understanding of the patient population served by the institution. Multiple viewpoints can also be an advantage in conflict resolution, especially when the conflict is related to diversity issues.

30. B: Sharing, supporting, and explaining the patient's point of view are activities that are consistent with advocacy. The remaining choices contribute to good professional practice but are not specifically related to the concept of advocacy.

Dear Adult CCRN Test Taker,

We would like to start by thanking you for purchasing this study guide for your Adult CCRN exam. We hope that we exceeded your expectations.

Our goal in creating this study guide was to cover all of the topics that you will see on the test. We also strove to make our practice questions as similar as possible to what you will encounter on test day. With that being said, if you found something that you feel was not up to your standards, please send us an email and let us know.

We would also like to let you know about other books in our catalog that may interest you.

CNOR

This can be found on Amazon: amazon.com/dp/1628456833

CEN

amazon.com/dp/1628457139

DTR

amazon.com/dp/1628454229

We have study guides in a wide variety of fields. If the one you are looking for isn't listed above, then try searching for it on Amazon or send us an email.

Thanks Again and Happy Testing!
Product Development Team
info@studyguideteam.com

FREE Test Taking Tips DVD Offer

To help us better serve you, we have developed a Test Taking Tips DVD that we would like to give you for FREE. **This DVD covers world-class test taking tips that you can use to be even more successful when you are taking your test.**

All that we ask is that you email us your feedback about your study guide. Please let us know what you thought about it – whether that is good, bad or indifferent.

To get your **FREE Test Taking Tips DVD**, email freedvd@studyguideteam.com with "FREE DVD" in the subject line and the following information in the body of the email:

     a. The title of your study guide.

     b. Your product rating on a scale of 1-5, with 5 being the highest rating.

     c. Your feedback about the study guide. What did you think of it?

     d. Your full name and shipping address to send your free DVD.

If you have any questions or concerns, please don't hesitate to contact us at freedvd@studyguideteam.com.

Thanks again!

Made in the USA
Middletown, DE
30 June 2020